Take Two Aspirin and Call Me By My Pronouns

Why Turning Doctors into Social Justice Warriors is Destroying American Medicine

STANLEY GOLDFARB, MD

BOMBARDIER

Published by Bombardier Books
An Imprint of Post Hill Press
ISBN: 978-1-64293-849-4
ISBN (eBook): 978-1-64293-850-0

Take Two Aspirin and Call Me By My Pronouns:
Why Turning Doctors into Social Justice Warriors is Destroying American Medicine
© 2022 by Stanley Goldfarb, MD
All Rights Reserved

Cover Design by Tiffani Shea
Interior Design by Yoni Limor

This is a work of nonfiction. All people, locations, events, and situations are portrayed to the best of the author's memory. This book contains advice and information relating to health care. It should be used to supplement rather than replace the advice of your doctor or another trained health professional. You are advised to consult your health professional with regard to matters related to your health, and in particular regarding matters that may require diagnosis or medical attention. All efforts have been made to assure the accuracy of the information in this book as of the date of publication. The publisher and the author disclaim liability for any medical outcomes that may occur as a result of applying the methods suggested in this book.

No part of this book may be reproduced, stored in a retrieval system, or transmitted by any means without the written permission of the author and publisher.

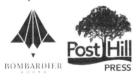

Post Hill Press
New York • Nashville
posthillpress.com

Published in the United States of America
1 2 3 4 5 6 7 8 9 10

Table of Contents

Chapter 1
Firestorm 1

Chapter 2
The Woke Insurrection 11

Chapter 3
First Among Unequals 25

Chapter 4
Admission Possible 33

Chapter 5
Dumbing Down 45

Chapter 6
The Color of Care 49

Chapter 7
Hypercritical Race Theory 61

Chapter 8
Not So Great Expectations 67

Chapter 9
What Price Atonement 81

Chapter 10
Unhelpful Changes 89

Chapter 11
The Ascendant Educational Class 99

Chapter 12
Remedial Med 101 107

Chapter 13
First, Seize the Media 113

Chapter 14
Confirmation Bias 125

Chapter 15
Saving the World 133

Chapter 16
Weaponizing Medicine 139

Chapter 17
Faking the Grade 147

Chapter 18
Millennial Coddling 157

Chapter 19
The Woke Assault on Merit 165

Chapter 20
Genes Matter 183

Chapter 21
When Black Doctors Doctored 191

Chapter 22
Back to the Future 203

About the Author 211

Chapter 1

Firestorm

American medicine is in trouble. The tenets of critical race theory (CRT) should concern not just every parent but every patient or potential patient, which is all of us. The CRT worldview threatens the quality of medical education and even of medical care. Educators at some leading health-care institutions have shown no more backbone than their counterparts at woke prep schools on Manhattan's Upper East Side. In health care, though, the stakes are higher. By abandoning traditional values such as treating all patients equally and recruiting the best and the brightest students, too many health educators have adopted a racialist agenda that will, if anything, aggravate health disparities and undermine the trust of patients of all races.

The quiet woke evolution of American medicine erupted in spring 2020 into a full-blown revolution. To protest the death of George Floyd in Minneapolis, thousands of doctors, nurses, and staff members across the nation emerged as instant social justice warriors, with many walking off the job in protest. At my institution, the University of Pennsylvania Perelman School of Medicine (hereafter, "Penn" or "Penn Medicine"), hundreds gathered in Philadelphia's Franklin Field to take an eight-minute-and-forty-six-second knee to honor the fallen George Floyd.

For years, activists had been primed for this moment. As Iboro Umana, an internal medicine resident at Penn, told *Penn Today*, "It's important to see so many people together addressing and realizing this is an issue and committing to working together to engage on this long process." Yes, it was a *long* process, the long march through the institutions. And now its foot soldiers were noisily marching through our medical schools and hospitals.

This symbolic gesture was the culmination of the growing woke movement in American health care. Public health leaders gave their blessing to massive, unmasked protests against supposed police brutality. They absurdly declared, "Racism is a public health crisis," and in the process made a joke of the field of public health. The medical profession had now positioned itself on the far side of the barricades.

Frightened at the thought of young radicals occupying their offices and undermining their highly successful clinical enterprises, too many leaders of American medicine signed on to the revolution. Their self-flagellation not only encouraged the radicals but also aggravated the distrust of the medical establishment in the Black community. What follows is an all too typical pronouncement from the CEO of Penn Medicine:

> There is no question we are at an inflection point on confronting racial injustice in our country, our city, and within our institution. The civil unrest that broke out this spring in response to the death of George Floyd—and so many Black people across the U.S. before him—brought to light the pervasive racism that is within all aspects of our culture, including medicine. Just as Penn Medicine leads in our field, we intend to lead as we more intentionally tackle racism, too.

So fearful was the CEO of seeming insensitive, he used Floyd's death to condemn the lifesaving work of his own institution. To do so, he had to ignore a seventy-year history of affirmative action initiatives. Worse, without evidence, he had to attribute the disparate outcomes between Black and White patients with chronic medical conditions—or even with COVID-19—to medical racism. This kind of positioning was widely echoed throughout the American health-care system. Its net effect was to alienate a large segment of the White public and sow further distrust of the medical establishment among Blacks.

I had grave concerns about the direction of American health care and medical education well before the woke eruption sparked by the pandemic and the George Floyd case. In September 2019, I wrote an op-ed for the *Wall Street Journal*. The editors mischievously titled it, "Take Two Aspirin and Call Me by My Pronouns." The tone of the article was considerably more sober than the headline, but for the easily triggered, the headline was enough. I can only imagine the hell I would have caught had I authored my *WSJ* op-ed in the wake of Floyd's death. It was bad enough in the fall of 2019.

Having spent my entire career practicing, teaching, and researching medicine, I was distressed to see medical school education lurch toward an increasing focus on social justice and other distractions that have zero to do with providing optimal care. Unfortunately, however, far too many medical professionals, especially young ones, care more about these issues than their responsibility to individual patients.

In a previous era, I argued, the commitment to caring for suffering patients was drilled into us aspiring young doctors. Sure, we were concerned with social problems as enlightened citizens, but we understood that the best use of our skills was to treat the sick. Now, led by a cadre of woke administrators who embraced the tenets of critical race theory, the medical establishment was committing itself to a misguided focus on anti-racism and equity in all aspects of the health-care system.

What bothered me the most was the ever-increasing urge to reject rigorous training in the scientific basis of medical care. Educators were championing instead a virtue signaling but ultimately impotent focus on the social issues du jour such as climate, gender equity, gun control, food deserts, and, most distressingly, race. The race obsession ran deepest. It was no fad. The new religion of "wokeism" demanded the acceptance of a crippling mythology that racism—or even White supremacy—was the cause of the very real disparities in health-care outcomes for Black communities.

These disparities have been recognized for many years, but their etiology has been correctly attributed to a complex mix of economic issues, cultural habits, and genetic predispositions. Now, however, medical journals were appeasing their critics by publishing medical researchers all too ready to blame physicians and institutional bias for the existence of such disparities.

To make their case, these researchers have scanned the evidence with the racial equivalent of Maslow's hammer. Said psychologist Abraham Maslow in 1966, "I suppose it is tempting, if the only tool you have is a hammer, to treat everything as if it were a nail." In this case, if your only tool is a magnifying glass that screens out everything but racism, then blows racism out of proportion, chances are you will find…racism. This field of research is, to say the least, shockingly corrupted by errors in study design, study interpretation, and yes, by the overt bias of certain investigators as well as of those authors who cite this research as background for their own investigations.

Despite the shoddiness of the research, the medical establishment decided that the only safe posture when accused of racism was to curl up in a ball and cry "Uncle!" To atone for past sins, educators embarked on a concerted effort to revise medical student and resident training to combat the "systemic racism" found in these flawed studies. For several years now, marginal students have been accepted into medical schools. Once accepted, they pass a curriculum whose aim is to assure that every student *will* pass. At the end, they will barely pass a series of watered-down licensure exams after extensive coaching and prep courses. From bottom to top, the system fails to weed out those who are performing poorly. The only people who will benefit are the trial lawyers reaping millions from malpractice cases.

Not willing to watch this systemic malpractice in silence, I spoke out. I decried the abandonment of our historical focus on training medical practitioners in the scientific basis of medicine. I rejected the ever-increasing commitment to topics best covered by schools of social work. And I dared to say so on the pages of the *Wall Street Journal.* For this apostasy, you would think I grabbed a tiki torch and marched through the streets of Philadelphia singing the praises of Robert E. Lee.

Even the enlightened educators at Penn were appalled that one of their own might dissent from their ever-increasing adoption of woke ideology. After my op-ed appeared, the authorities promptly sought to unruffle the feathers of our easily ruffled students:

> Please know that the views expressed by Dr. Goldfarb in his column reflect his personal opinions and do not reflect the values of the Perelman School of Medicine. We deeply value inclusion and diversity as fundamental to effective health care delivery, creativity, discovery, and life-long learning. We are committed to ensuring a rigorous and comprehensive medical education that includes examination of the many social and cultural issues that influence health, from violence within communities to changes in the environment around us.

Without intending, the drafters of this apology confirmed my thesis. Their statement nicely captured the nonsense that is consuming medical education and threatening the quality of medical care in the United States. In truth, "inclusion and diversity" do not rank high on the list of patient concerns when they are about to undergo surgery. As the anesthesia takes hold, the one thing patients do "deeply value" is competence.

Even less thrilled with my opinion were the Twitter warriors, many of them physicians. As I learned, the term of art for those who endorse traditional medical education is "asshole." "Stanley Goldfarb not only makes a terrible argument—and is arguably an asshole for his comments—but he's dead wrong," tweeted Nicholas Evans[1], an associate professor at the University of Massachusetts. "We know issues of justice matter to patient care, and ultimately to patient outcomes."

Just stop for a moment and ask yourself how knowing some social justice cliché improves the cardiac function of a patient suffering from shortness of breath or the blood pressure of a patient in shock due to a severe infection. As I have discovered, social justice warriors are simply unwilling to engage in self-examination or acknowledge their impotence in altering social conditions.

Ryan Marino, a self-described "human doctor," piled on. "Stanley Goldfarb is the latest asshole to try to tell doctors to 'stay in their lane,'" wrote Marino. "Well, Dr. Goldfarb is a *former* dean, and I'm happy to report that the future of medicine is ready to forget all about people like him while we remember to make ALL our patients' lives better."[2]

One entity called "Progressive Doctors" tweeted, "Whining, reactionary, white, male doctors want medicine depoliticized of the left. So that they can be political themselves." To prove I was a reactionary, this bunch went to the trouble of finding my political donations and posting them online. The radical right firebrands

---

1. Nicholas G. Evans, "Stanley Goldfarb not only makes a terrible argument—and is arguably an asshole for his comments—but he's dead wrong. We know issues of justice matter to patient care, and ultimately to patient outcomes," Twitter, September 15, 2019, https://twitter.com/neva9257/status/1173023731201060865.
2. Ryan Marino, "Stanley Goldfarb is the latest asshole to try to tell doctors to 'stay in their lane.' Well, Dr. Goldfarb is a *former* dean, and I'm happy to report that the future of medicine is ready to forget all about people like him while we remember to make ALL our patients' lives better," Twitter, September 13, 2019, https://twitter.com/RyanMarino/status/1172491117021057026.

I had supported included John McCain, Mitt Romney, Arlen Specter, and John Hickenlooper, a Democrat. God only knows what would have happened to me had they unearthed a donation to Donald Trump.[3]

Not to be left out of the critics' circle was the *New England Journal of Medicine*, arguably the most authoritative medical journal. As exhibit one, let me cite an article by Dr. Paul Farmer and colleagues—for simplicity's sake, the "Farmer docs." Farmer was chair of the Department of Global Health and Social Medicine at Harvard Medical School, among other titles. Writing in the *New England Journal of Medicine* in 2020, the Farmer docs directly attacked me for arguing that physicians have no particular ability to improve social conditions and should remain focused on the care of individual patients:

> In a 2019 op-ed in the Wall Street Journal entitled "Take Two Aspirin and Call Me by My Pronouns," former University of Pennsylvania Dean of Medical Education Stanley Goldfarb echoed a dismissal that some physicians have been voicing for decades. Why should medical training focus on social factors, Goldfarb asked, when medicine's purpose is to cure individual patients? His essay assumed that one can effectively cure patients while ignoring the world in which they live. Unfortunately, that is an empirically untenable position.

Of course, I never recommended that doctors "ignore" the world in which patients live. The Farmer docs went on to provide the true motive for their rebuttal. They were not subtle:

---

[3]. Progressive Doctors, "Whining, reactionary, white, male doctors want medicine depoliticized of the left. So that they can be political themselves," Twitter, September 15, 2019, https://twitter.com/progressiveMDs/status/1173240793282355202.

> Physicians risk misdiagnosis when we fail to take social structures into account or misattribute their effects to biologic mechanisms or individual behaviors. A well-recognized example of large-scale misdiagnosis involves the multiple, intertwined epidemics of chronic disease that are related to housing and food insecurity in low-income neighborhoods. These diseases — including diabetes, heart disease, obesity, asthma, mood and anxiety disorders, and substance use disorder — cluster together zoogeographically into what have been termed "syndemics." […] Syndemics are related to certain neighborhoods' unstable housing and dearth of healthy food, which reflect a history of institutional racism — including redlining — and stark socioeconomic inequalities produced by capitalism.

The end of the statement gives the game away. "Capitalism" is apparently the cause of disease, and capitalism's elimination would appear to be the cure envisioned by Farmer et al. This is not medicine; it is political ideology, propaganda even. It assumes that medical students and trainees would do well to keep a copy of *Das Kapital* on their bookshelves alongside, say, Netter's *Atlas of Human Anatomy* or Harrison's *Principles of Internal Medicine*.

Although a seeming expert on everything else, Karl Marx knew enough to keep his nose out of medicine. Physicians in training should return the favor and keep their noses out of Marx. This kind of ideological nonsense does not belong in medical school curricula. And yet, it is becoming a major educational focus of most medical schools in the United States.

In their rush to condemn me, these critics refuse to acknowledge the contemporary state of American medicine. Although medical care in the United States is often very good, it is not consistently very good. In a landmark analysis, Dr. Betsy Williams of Rush Medical College reported that between 6 and 12 percent of physicians perform in an "unsatisfactory" manner. A study by the VA health system found that even by the VA's standards, some 40 percent of the nonveteran public was receiving suboptimal care for a variety of clinical conditions such as hypertension, diabetes, and coronary artery disease. These statistics should frighten every American. They call for improved physician training, not for indoctrination into progressive political causes.

I have personally been fortunate to work with very capable colleagues at my school and hospital, a highly regarded medical school and health-care system, but I have certainly worked with students who managed to pass through a less than rigorous assessment system in medical school despite disciplinary actions, suspensions, and near dismissals. This decline in standards is not unique to Penn but is rampant in medical schools across the nation. There is no justification for passing even one underperforming, "dyscompetent" student, yet perhaps as many as 3 to 5 percent of all med school graduates do not deserve the title "doctor." Even of greater concern, many more have a deficient grasp of the scientific basis of medical care.

In the near future, this situation will only get worse. Those who muster under the banner of social justice feel empowered to do whatever they want to have their agendas enacted. Those agendas will not focus on individual merit, equal opportunity, and liberty. They will be racist in the name of "anti-racism," and they will eschew all marks of academic and professional achievement in the name of equity. Those who oppose this agenda will be shoved aside, if not out the door.

To prevent this from happening, I have expanded my "two aspirin" thesis into a book. My goal is to inspire my fellow assholes to go full Howard Beale and shout from the rooftops, "I'm as mad as hell, and I'm not going to take this anymore."

Chapter 2

The Woke Insurrection

Before the spring of George Floyd and COVID-19, few of us were awake to the silent woke coup on our institutions, the medical establishment most ominously. The dictionary defines the word *woke* as "alert to injustice in society, especially racism." This definition is much too benign. In real life, as we saw that spring, "woke" is a scarier condition. The woke movement, as it has evolved on our shores, has a hard edge to it. It strikes me as an uneasy mix of the American New Left and the Chinese Red Guard. Woke insurrectionists have muscled their way into every major American institution, most pervasively the education establishment. Their strengths are their passion, their indifference to the truth, and their reckless urge to slander their opponents.

"If people were to understand that racism, and all of the social and political and economic inequalities that racism creates, ultimately harms people's health," pediatrician Dr. Rhea Boyd told *Time* magazine in support of the COVID-19-defying protests by medical professionals, they would see that "protest is a profound public health intervention, because it allows us to finally address and end forms of inequality."

Boyd was not an outlier. "Risking coronavirus pales in comparison to all the other ways we can die," added Dr. Dorothy Charles, a family medicine resident and organizer of the group White Coats for Black Lives. "Addressing the root causes [of racial inequality] is more imperative at this point than staying at home."[4] Although admitting that each day of protest could lead to as many as three thousand new coronavirus infections, virology researcher Trevor Bedford thought the risks were worth it. "The harms of systemic racism are real and utterly pernicious," Bedford tweeted. "The hope is that the protests may lead to lasting reform."

These quotes capture the syllogistic fallacy of the social justice movement: Structural racism has made people of color more susceptible to dying from COVID-19; the only way to end racism is to protest; the protests will lead to better health outcomes. But there is never a path from the protests to a better outcome. Not only did the protests spread COVID-19, but they also spread anxiety about the admittedly racist medical establishment. As will become increasingly clear, the movement matters more to its movers and shakers than does the health of the people they pretend to care about.

These twin events—the pandemic and the protests—served to soften any resistance to an AMA master plan first conceived in 2018 and released in 2021, "Organizational Strategic Plan to Embed Racial Justice and Advance Health Equity, 2021–2023." As the nation's largest professional association of physicians, the American Medical Association has serious clout. By putting its imprimatur on this Orwellian eighty-six-page document, AMA leadership is dictating the future of American health care. That future is a dim one. Unlike other social justice programs, this program is lethal. It will tangibly reduce the quality of medical care, and almost every American will suffer its side effects. The AMA may call itself "a unifying voice," but it unifies through coercion. Many physicians no more welcome the AMA's master

---

4. Jamie Ducharme, "'Protest Is a Profound Public Health Intervention,'" *Time*, June 10, 2020, https://time.com/5848212/doctors-supporting-protests/.

plan "for equity and justice in medicine" than they would an unmarked package from Wuhan, China, but they understandably fear to speak out.

The authors of the master plan fear little. They are certainly not afraid to bite the hand that feeds them. Indeed, they treat the AMA the way Nelson Mandela treated the outgoing apartheid leadership of South Africa but without Mandela's sense of mercy and forgiveness. Among the "five strategic approaches to advance equity and justice" is this gem, "Foster truth, racial healing, reconciliation and transformation for the AMA's past." America's physicians have created the best and fairest health-care system in the world. They have doubled the American life span in a century. They have created the lion's share of lifesaving drugs and technologies used worldwide. And yet the master plan authors want them to atone for their "past." The tone of the document is perhaps best captured in a quote, centered and emboldened, from the aforementioned Dr. Rhea Boyd:

> The truth is, our nation's investment in racism, capitalism, and white supremacy shredded our safety net, almost cost us our democracy, and stole many of our loved ones' lives. In the middle of our loneliest year, our dependence on each other—for public education, public health, public utilities, and public recreation—was the truth buried beneath our pain. As we begin to slowly emerge from the depths of this plague, how we make sense of that truth will determine our future.

This is the language of a demagogue, an angry and delusional one. Stand in the woke insurrection's way, and you can bank on being called a racist, sexist, homophobe, science denier, fat-shamer. The AMA's racial hectoring is mild compared to that of the much too influential outfit, White Coats for Black Lives (WC4BL). Its mission statement, "Our Vision and Values," published in June 2021, reads like a manifesto from the Weather Underground. "Our job is two-fold," its authors insist. The first job, no small one, involves "dismantling dominant, exploitative systems in the United States, which are largely reliant on anti-Black racism, colonialism, cisheteropatriarchy, white supremacy, and capitalism." Having eliminated cisheteropatriarchy, whatever that is, the White Coats move on to their second job. This job, of course, would be rendered impossible if they succeeded at the first, namely "rebuilding a future that supports the health and well-being of marginalized communities."[5] What is scary is just how seriously the medical establishment takes WC4BL. The organization has chapters at more than seventy medical schools across the country, including many of the more prestigious. Fail to yield to the White Coats and their allies, and these clueless young Jacobins will lustily call for your head. Liberals, who have largely managed academia for the last half century, are too eager to pacify their radical allies to resist.

Harvard Medical School (HMS) is a case in point. In April 2021, HMS announced the launch of a task force to address racism. Although it may not be apparent to outsiders, Harvard, according to its dean for medical education, Edward Hundert, has "a history of white supremacist culture." The claim that American medical schools, particularly the most prestigious medical schools, are nests of white supremacy is mind-bogglingly absurd. For a half century or longer, these schools have been at the forefront of affirmative action programs, minority hiring initiatives, and special programs for recruiting and supporting minority students and faculty. In their affiliated urban hospitals, they have provided exemplary care to the Black community. Yet the self-denigration is unabated.

---

5. "Our Vision and Values," White Coats for Black Lives, June 25, 2021, https://whitecoats4blacklives.org/wp-content/uploads/2021/07/WC4BL_Vision_Document_1_.pdf.

White supremacy apparently manifests itself, says Dean Hundert, in that the retention rate for White students at HMS is higher than it is for Black and other "underrepresented" students. "We have to hold that [disparity] up, address it, and work on it," said the obviously cowed dean. In future chapters, I will address what "work on it" means for the health of the average patient. The reader can well imagine.

To be sure, there is scarcely an educational institution in America—from preschool to medical school—that has not been invaded by the woke. Once inside an institution, they camp out in every available school and department, heading up new and pointless programs titled "diversity," "inclusivity," "equity," or some combination of the above. According to a report by the Heritage Foundation, the University of Michigan has some 163 officers dedicated to "diversity, equity, and/or inclusivity."

We have tolerated this nonsense because it does not seem to affect us. Medical schools are different…lives are at stake. As shall be seen, the woke obsession with gender, ethnicity, sexual orientation, climate, guns, income inequality, and especially with race has infected every nook and cranny of the medical education process—from admission to grading to graduating to internships to honor societies to publications to diagnosing patients. In that this infection shows consistent symptoms wherever it roots, my diagnosis will inevitably seem a bit repetitive. Please bear with me if it does. Americans need to understand the depth of the rot and the difficulty of excising it.

Make no mistake: These trends embody the worst of wokeism. They are accelerating throughout American medicine and will lead to outcomes detrimental to the health care of even the patients the movement claims to serve. Activists call for abandoning meritocracy, academic rigor, selectivity in recruitment, and color-blind medicine. It is one thing for the Princeton classics department to abandon its Latin requirement for classics majors. It is quite another thing for Harvard Med to cut training time in biochemistry and pharmacology for future doctors. After all, no one dies if the classics major cannot conjugate *morior*.

Like many revolutionary movements, this one began as something small and seemingly harmless. The philosophical origins of the idea that physicians are responsible for correcting inequities in health status among different communities arose in the years following World War II and gained ground in the ensuing decades. Medical ethicists and sociologists proposed this idea in an intellectual milieu favorable to socialist policies. Among the more influential thinkers in this proto-Marxist school was Ivan Illich, an Austrian immigrant and Roman Catholic priest. His 1974 book, *Medical Nemesis*, provided a philosophical foundation for a communitarian approach to health care.

Illich proposed that health care was erroneously focused on eradicating pain and sickness, even death. Rather, he argued that physicians did more harm than good in their focused treatment of individual patients. He popularized the word "iatrogenesis"—meaning "physician-generated illness"—and used it to suggest that physicians intervene in their patient's health too aggressively and often mistakenly. Illich disdained the growth of medical technology and coined the term "medicalization" to describe the commercial aspects of medical care he loathed. Rejecting the rush to high-tech medicine, he favored an emphasis on nutrition and social justice to maintain the health of the community.

Illich's ideas were widely debated in the medical community and elicited strong counter opinions. But his concepts resonated among socially conscious physicians and paved the way for the current initiatives to integrate social justice into the practice of medicine and to prepare medical students to be advocates for social activism.

In his time, Illich faced considerable resistance. Influential physicians such as Edmund Pellegrino and Donald Seldin objected to Illich's formulation. An influential medical ethicist, Dr. Pellegrino confronted the dilemma faced by physicians over whether their focus should be on caring for individual patients or on trying to improve the health status of a community. Given limited resources, Pellegrino believed that the physician's primary responsibility was to the individual patient. He was among those physicians who preferred that investments be channeled into high technology and care for sick patients. This excerpt from a 1980 essay summarizes Pellegrino's position:

> The physician…promises that all his special skill and competence will be put at the service of the patient. The prime focus of all the physician's activity is the good of the person who presents himself here and now—not some distant patient who may be more worthy, not the good of society or the family, and certainly not the good of the physician or the institution he may serve.

This position clearly conflicts with the idea that physicians become advocates for social justice. All of a physician's professional effort, Pellegrino believed, must be focused on the care of the individual patient.

Dr. Donald Seldin, an influential academic physician—he founded the University of Texas Southwestern Medical Center and Medical School, home to several Nobel Prize winners—was even more adamant about the need to focus on the individual patient. As a witness at the Nuremberg war crime trials, Seldin invoked the horror of Nazi medical experimentations as the ultimate corruption of medical ethics. He attributed this deviation to physicians whose social activism led them into the arms of the Third Reich. He saw a danger in a modern medical establishment already straying from its historic focus on patient care. As he wrote in his seminal address to the Association of American Physicians in 1981:

> [...] I shall argue that medicine is a very narrow discipline. Its goals may be defined as the relief of pain, the prevention of disability, and the postponement of death by the application of the theoretical knowledge incorporated in medical science to individual patients.

Two understandings flowed from this definition. One was that although medicine was a "comparatively weak scientific discipline," it nonetheless remained a powerful tool to alleviate suffering and prolong life. The second, less helpful consequence was the tendency to elevate physicians to a priestly caste and "construe all sorts of human problems as medical problems." Wrote Seldin:

> This medicalization of human experience leads to an enormous hypertrophy of personnel and facilities, massive financial expenditures, and perhaps most tragic of all, frustration and disillusionment when medical intervention fails to eventuate in tranquility, quiescence, and happiness.

Despite these powerful statements affirming the centrality of the care of individual patients in a physician's professional life, the idea that physicians should involve themselves in social issues continued to metastasize. The 1978 Alma-Alta Declaration produced by the World Health Organization (WHO) showed the movement going international. Primary health care, from the WHO's perspective, "addresses the main health problems in the community, providing promotive, preventive, curative and rehabilitative services accordingly." The role of the physician in this scenario included the following:

> [...] education concerning prevailing health problems and the methods of preventing

and controlling them; promotion of food supply and proper nutrition; an adequate supply of safe water and basic sanitation; maternal and child health care, including family planning; immunization against the major infectious diseases; prevention and control of locally endemic diseases; appropriate treatment of common diseases and injuries; and provision of essential drugs.

The WHO's declaration springs from Illich's concepts of the role of medical care as a social activity. Given the demands on the physician's time in this busy scenario, we have to wonder when that physician might actually see a patient.

By the turn of the century, the die had been cast, and it took on a particularly American veneer. In August 2002, Dr. Alan Nelson, past president of the American Medical Association, made a game-changing speech to the Institute of Medicine of the National Academy of Sciences. He called on his fellow physicians to address racial and ethnic disparities in health care. Fair enough. He attributed the generally poor outcomes and shorter life expectancy for Black patients to the social conditions that plague inner-city Black communities. Again, fair enough.

Nelson then entered uncharted waters. He raised the specter that racial bias in the delivery of health care just might contribute to the poor outcomes. Before wading in too deep, however, he was careful to point out that much study was necessary before validating this possibility. Twenty years later, despite considerable study, the medical community is no closer to consensus on the reason for disparate outcomes than when Nelson made his clarion call.

The attack piece by Paul Farmer and colleagues referred to earlier nicely illustrates the illogic of the assertion that to understand social issues is as important for a doctor as to understand the biologic basis of disease. "When chronic conditions are viewed as solely biologic or behavioral malfunction," the Farmer docs insisted, "the diagnosis misses the true causes, and often, misdiagnosis leads to ineffective treatments." This argument might have swayed me if they had provided a single example of a physician whose knowledge of the patient's social conditions—or lack thereof—had made the slightest difference in the patient's clinical outcome.

One case the Farmer docs cite is that of a man who entered the emergency department of a hospital complaining of abdominal pain. This case was part of a series on "Case Studies in Social Medicine" published in the *New England Journal of Medicine* in 2018. Upon further questioning and examination, it turned out that the patient was a biological female in the process of gender transition and was pregnant. I know, a tricky business. The Farmer docs argued that medical students needed an extended educational program in the psychological issues associated with transgender patients to treat the patient.

You do not need to be an ob-gyn physician to figure this one out, and you don't need coursework in transgender studies to tell a biological female from a biological male. The diagnosis of pregnancy is *always* considered when a biological woman enters with abdominal pain. A physical exam and a history would have done the trick. The immediate problem was clinical. The hand-holding could come after the mother—yes, mother—and baby were safe.

If anything, this particular case undermines the idea that students need to have a deep understanding of the social issues surrounding gender—but it does reinforce the importance of knowing how to do a complete physical examination. This includes an exam of the patient's genitalia. The ER is no place to be coy. Yes, transgender patients do have specific medical issues that require practitioner familiarity. Beyond having that knowledge, however, physicians cannot prevent violence against transgender individuals or alter society's perceptions of them in any meaningful way. Again, Farmer and colleagues failed to identify the flaws in my argument that extensive training in social determinants of health would not have mattered in this patient's care.

Parenthetically, Penn has an extensive curriculum on the medical needs of transgender subjects that I strongly supported. There is no question that there are major psychological problems associated with gender transition. But immersing the students in those social and psychological issues subtracts from the time spent on medical training.

A second case in the series cited by the Farmer docs concerns a child living in rural Mexico who presented with severe pneumonia. An American physician working in that area found that the child's family was very poor and that the child was undernourished. The authors of the *New England Journal of Medicine* article cited the case to show how poverty can affect health. Physicians, they argued, should learn the signs and symptoms of malnutrition and report them to social services when available.

Fair enough. In rural Mexico, however, American physicians have little agency. The authors describe how the physician attempted to teach the local residents how to farm. The crops failed. He then attempted to introduce livestock into the community to improve nutrition, but this project failed too. The authors settled on the theory that food shortages in the community stemmed from a centuries-old feudal system about which they could do nothing. This is the follow-up from the case:

> In the months following his pneumonia treatment, Dr. R.'s patient continued to be chronically malnourished. But the malnutrition-program participants remained dedicated to improving children's lives, though they have, to date, achieved only minor improvements in nutritional outcomes.

These doctors are no doubt to be congratulated for their discovery of widespread malnutrition due to conditions of rural poverty that have been endemic throughout the world for thousands of years. These problems preceded the advent of capitalism and are unfortunately not likely to be solved by it any time soon.

The bottom line here seems to be that farming is best left to farmers and medicine to doctors. The article brutally proves the pointlessness of physicians trying to solve social problems that are beyond their power to change and for which they have no expertise or training. Yet, the Farmer docs highlight this case as an example of how social consciousness can improve health. What this community needed was a competent Peace Corps volunteer, not a physician turned social worker.

The absence of evidence did not discourage Farmer and colleagues from pushing their Marxist ideas. They insist that indoctrinating medical students in soft-core Marxist theory and devoting major portions of their time to social issues is a good and necessary thing:

> Clinicians are uniquely positioned to respond to the social, political, and economic structures affecting our patients' health. If we fail to do so, we risk misdiagnosis, mistreatment, and iatrogenic harm. We are convinced that undergraduate, graduate, and continuing medical education in structural competency and other social medicine frameworks can be used to train clinicians who will thrive while effectively confronting the health problems caused by inequitable social structures.

As a reminder, "iatrogenic" refers to medical treatment that makes the patient worse. Nothing new here. For the last few thousand years, doctors have been schooled in the idea, "First, do no harm." The best way to "do no harm" is to know how to do good medicine. The more time spent on sowing crops or social work, the less time will be spent on patient care.

Farmer and his colleagues were hardly the only critics I faced in response to my article. Something called "MedTwitter" exploded with attacks on my position. Almost all the critics discounted my thesis, but not one provided an example in which a physician's delving into community organizing improved clinical outcomes.

There was, however, a great deal of virtue signaling, particularly by recent medical school graduates. One former Penn student, Dr. Crystal Zheng, decided that my criticism of the medical school curriculum required an open letter to me by one hundred fifty medical school alumni proposing that I had betrayed them by not following the party line.

The harassment escalated. It always does. In the eyes of the true believer, those who challenge the idea of systemic racism might as well exchange their white lab coats for white sheets. According to the believers, social justice skeptics have no business guiding young minds.

There is no denying that skeptics like me are on the run, and the woke are in command. Their dominance in medical schools and academic medical centers is well established. We now have a medical school curriculum steeped in ideas that make much more sense in an undeveloped country than in a developed one. Sensible or not, we are aggressively moving to transform the physician workforce into a woke advocacy corps for social justice issues.

Researchers at the University of Oregon, writing in the journal of *Academic Medicine* in 2021, surveyed the curricula of 122 medical schools and found that more than half had a *required* course that covered elements of advocacy. Of the 112 schools that published their elective course descriptions online, two-thirds offered elective courses on advocacy. On average, schools offered both required and elective courses on various advocacy topics. I haven't read them all, but I am going to guess those advocacy issues do not include the protection of life, liberty, or the pursuit of happiness.

Chapter 3

First Among Unequals

The esteemed Greek physician Hippocrates was born some two thousand four hundred years before Penn Medicine and other medical schools decided they had an obligation to change the world. If Hippocrates protested the injustices of his day, we do not know about it. What we do know is that he practiced medicine at a higher level than the world had yet seen. To this day, the oath attributed to Hippocrates bears reading. "I will use those dietary regimens which will benefit my patients according to my greatest ability and judgment, and I will do no harm or injustice to them," wrote Hippocrates. "Neither will I administer a poison to anybody when asked to do so, nor will I suggest such a course. Similarly I will not give to a woman a pessary to cause abortion. But I will keep pure and holy both my life and my art."

In the oath, Hippocrates acknowledges the existence of slavery. "Into whatsoever houses I enter, I will enter to help the sick, and I will abstain from all intentional wrong-doing and harm, especially from abusing the bodies of man or woman, bond or free." The doctor's obligation to the bonded servants was not to free them—that was impossible—but to treat them with the same care as he would their masters.

In sum, the traditional Hippocratic oath bound physicians to heal the sick through dedication to ethical care and professionalism. It spoke nothing about venturing into the social justice arena with all its inherent conflicts between various political and philosophical worldviews.

Yet, in America today, too many med students and physicians have less desire "to help the sick" than to cure what they see as society's ills. And although it may not be "intentional," there is no denying that the result of their efforts amounts to "wrongdoing and harm." The social ill they see as most toxic is racism. Despite massive evidence to the contrary, many believe the disease has mutated into "White supremacy."

The issue of race drives the progressive movement. If proof were needed, the George Floyd protests during the summer of 2020 provided it. All the other allegedly "marginalized" groups that make up the "intersectional" coalition understood they were just along for the ride. Race was the engine of change. It is the one issue that scares even well-intentioned educators into betraying the liberal principles they hold dear.

Not surprisingly, Harvard Medical School has been leading the movement toward illiberalism. The medical school website has several links to progressive organizations, including those cheerleaders for Venezuelan poverty and Cuban oppression, Black Lives Matter. The Winter 2021 issue of the school's magazine, *Harvard Medicine*, features Dr. Andrea Reid, Harvard's chief guru of multiculturalism, discussing "race-based medicine."

Echoing the Association of American Medical Colleges' position on racism, Reid does her best to indict the physician workforce for racist behavior. She's not invoking historical racism but racism in the here and now. Focusing on the subject of pain treatment, Reid makes the bizarre argument that physicians shortchange Black patients, believing them inherently less sensitive to pain than White patients.

Like so many researchers looking through Maslow's magnifying glass, Reid either misquotes, misinterprets, or deliberately distorts the existing studies to sustain the racism narrative. The problem of treating pain in any patient is complex. All doctors know this. Proper treatment requires an individual approach to each patient. The literature on this subject is extensive, but the evidence that Black patients are consistently undertreated for pain is sketchy at best.

For example, a careful study from the emergency department of Saint Louis University School of Medicine showed that Black patients and White patients received the same opioid analgesics when they suffered from fractured long bones or had migraine headaches. Fewer Black patients with back pain were prescribed opioids, but they received comparable amounts of other analgesics when compared to White patients.

This is a complex subject. The literature on this topic suggests that patient demands, physician training in pain management, and concern about administering opioid analgesics all may influence physician decisions. Certainly, the physicians in St. Louis were hardly ignoring any pain in their Black patients. Moreover, when the study assessed how Black physicians at the school treated pain in Black and White patients, it found no real difference in their use of opioid analgesics compared to that of White physicians. Unclear, too, was whether White patients were disproportionately receiving inappropriate pain medicine like Oxycontin. The assumption is that Black patients receive less quality care when, in fact, it is the White patients who are more likely to be treated inappropriately with opioids.

Harvard's Dr. Reid has little use for contrary evidence. Reid is adamant that medical workers cling to biases about the nervous system of Black patients. These biases, she argues, contribute to disparate outcomes in the treatment of pain. To prove this contention, she relied on a 2016 study in the prestigious journal, *Proceedings of the National Academy of Sciences* (*PNAS*). This study surveyed University of Virginia medical students on their attitudes about the biologic characteristics of Black and White patients. She highlighted a question in the survey about pain perception. As she interpreted the results, 50 percent of medical students thought, erroneously, that Black patients have fewer nerve endings than White patients and therefore would perceive less pain. This idea, she surmised, explained why the literature suggests differential treatment patterns.

To support her thesis, however, she ignores crucial information. The only medical students who felt that Black patients had different neural characteristics were first- and second-year students. They almost certainly had not yet had courses in neurology or pain management. To include them in a survey to assess mature health-care providers' beliefs on any topic is ludicrous. When third-year students were queried, none endorsed the spurious idea about "Black nerve endings." By their third year, the students had completed their preclinical coursework and engaged in clinical medicine.

If anything, this study showed the exact opposite of Reid's claim about physician bias in medical care for Black patients. The University of Virginia School of Medicine succeeded quite nicely in correctly educating students about nerve endings in Black patients. Had the school squandered the students' time inculcating racialist views, the students might not have learned as much as they did. Yet, Dr. Reid and others misrepresent this study as the foundation for their accusation of racism on the part of physicians and trainees and bias about the physical characteristics of Black patients.

It is distressing to note that this *PNAS* article has been cited in one hundred and thirty-five other articles in the medical literature as evidence of medical racism. One can be all but certain that the authors of these articles neglect the subtleties of the original and, like Dr. Reid, misuse the study to support the accusation of physician bias.

For example, Dr. Kavita Algu cites the Virginia study in an article published in 2021 in the journal *eClinicalMedicine*. There is no subtlety in her title: "Denied the right to comfort: Racial inequities in palliative care provision" as evidence of medical racism. Dr. Algu misrepresents the *PNAS* article to suggest that Black patients are denied treatment for pain although the article has nothing to do with the actual treatment. From reading it, she somehow concludes, "For example, a false belief that people who are Black feel less pain was created as a tool of oppression and slavery. Its legacy continues, and Black adults and children still endure inadequate treatment of their pain." Where did this mishmash of bad history and worse logic come from?

Most readers of Dr. Algu's paper and the other hundred-plus articles citing the *PNAS* paper will not access the original reference and find the distortion, one that is all too commonplace in the literature on health-care disparities and the role of physician bias.

Dr. Reid's idea of a medical establishment infected with structural racism and her passion for physician advocacy is not unusual. They dominate contemporary medical education. They are mutually reinforcing concepts, and they are both terribly flawed. The former relies on a superficial, biased, and often mistaken assessment of the medical literature on disparate health outcomes. The latter is the result of a utopian and wholly unrealistic conception of the appropriateness and efficacy of a physician advocacy corps for social issues. A new breed of physician educators endorses both these mistaken ideas. Steeped in progressive educational theories, these educators are committing their institutions to unworkable solutions to social ills and the radical transformation of medical education.

A recent article in the prestigious medical journal, *The Lancet*, defines structural racism as the "totality of ways in which societies foster racial discrimination through mutually reinforcing systems of housing, education, employment, earnings, benefits, credit, media, health care, and criminal justice." The authors' solution to structural racism is, in part, an extensive training program for medical students and others.

The leaders of American academic medicine justify widespread commitments to social justice training based on the concept of systemic racism. This initiative only makes sense if medical care itself is riddled with racism. If the basis for "structural racism" is the array of social inequalities found in minority communities, the care patients receive in physicians' offices and the hospital cannot solve those problems.

Nonetheless, politicians, the popular press, and even leaders of medicine such as the deans of Harvard Medical School and the Perelman School at Penn have decreed that racism in medical care itself needs to be rooted out. But carefully examining the evidence for widespread racism in medical care shows that evidence to be slight. Again, while social ills might contribute to poor health, the remedy for social ills is not found in the health-care system nor the professional activities of physicians.

Current criticisms of the health-care system by activists assume that poor health outcomes in African American communities are in large part attributable to poor medical care. If this were true, then an initiative to purge all the racist tendencies in physicians and a curriculum to teach medical students more about bias and discrimination would make complete sense. But the assumption is false. Solving a problem that doesn't exist will be a disastrous waste of time and resources. Bias workshops, symposia featuring anti-racist speakers, hiring practices that focus more and more on a person's skin color, and another five hours a week for medical students in racial justice classes will all further compromise the quality of medical education and, ultimately, the American health-care system.

What is curious about the AMA master plan discussed earlier is that when the authors speak of "intended outcomes," they are referring not to the health of minority communities but the health of their "brand." I wish I were kidding. What follows are the variables they are keen to measure:[6]

---

6. These variables are directly quoted from the AMA's "Organizational Strategic Plan to Embed Racial Justice and Advance Health Equity," 2021–2023, https://www.ama-assn.org/system/files/2021-05/ama-equity-strategic-plan.pdf.

- *Health Equity (i.e., as a general metric in medicine, in advocacy, in policy)

- *Partnerships and sharing power (i.e., trust, reciprocity, power sharing)

- *Diversity, equity and inclusion (i.e., AMA workforce, membership and medicine)

- *Cultural shift (i.e., attitudes, behaviors and policies)

- *Truth, racial healing, reconciliation and transformation (i.e., qualitative interviews to understand extent of past harm and progress towards healing, reconciliation and transformation across different sectors of health care and public health)

- *Impact (i.e., mission, audience reach, membership and brand)

Missing from the AMA master plan is any evidence that traces the disparity in medical outcomes to poor medical care, let alone to care rendered poor by the racism of the physicians or the system. To justify radical changes in medical education, the evidence should be overwhelming. It is not.

Glenn Loury, an African American public intellectual and a professor at Brown University, has criticized the notion of structural racism as a catchall explanation for the disparate circumstances of African Americans. In his essay, "Unspeakable Truths about Racial Inequality in America," Loury writes:

> Users don't even pretend to offer evidence-based arguments beyond citing the fact of the racial disparity itself. The "structural racism" argument seldom goes into cause

and effect. Rather, it asserts shadowy causes that are never fully specified, let alone demonstrated. We are all just supposed to know that it's the fault of something called "structural racism," abetted by an environment of "white privilege," furthered by an ideology of "white supremacy" that purportedly characterizes our society. It explains everything.

Loury goes on to confront those social critics who refuse to acknowledge a component of individual agency in explaining disparate social outcomes. As he notes, those critics also tend to ignore the effect of self-destructive behaviors. In denying African Americans the will to shape their own futures, and only African Americans, the social justice activists practice a more profound racism than any of the people they criticize.

Chapter 4

Admission Possible

So much of what has deformed medical education can be traced to one simple fact: There are fewer Black doctors than equity advocates think there ought to be. These advocates often use the acronyms "URM" or "UIM"—meaning "underrepresented in medicine"—to suggest that there is widespread discrimination against minorities, but the real issue has always been and continues to be the number of practicing Black doctors.

The advocates' concern is not without merit. In 1996, when Drs. Herbert Nickens and Jordan Cohen, the latter then president of the Association of American Medical Colleges (AAMC), made the case for racial diversity in a much-cited essay, African Americans comprised less than 2 percent of medical school matriculants. At the time, Blacks made up about 13 percent of the American population.[7]

In the article, the authors acknowledged that the medical community had been trying aggressively to right historic wrongs since the 1960s and had "dramatic" success, at least initially. Despite the best efforts of the medical establishment, however, the numbers soon flatlined. Like the authors of the AMA master plan,

---

7. Herbert Nickens and Jordan Cohen, "On Affirmative Action," *The Journal of the American Medical Association* (February 21, 1996), https://jamanetwork.com/journals/jama/article-abstract/396923.

Cohen and Nickens seemed more interested in proving that affirmative action could "work" than they did in questioning whether it improved the health outcome of minority patients.

The authors outlined several reasons for redoubling the effort to increase the admission of Black students to medical school. First, they endorsed the progressive idea of equity. To break down barriers to admission meant little to Progressives if Black students were still proportionately underrepresented.

Cohen and Nickens also argued that since Black physicians have a greater tendency to practice in Black communities, medical schools should produce more Black physicians to meet physician demand in so-called medically underserved areas (MUAs). As a corollary point, they argued that Black physicians could do a better job of providing care to Black patients through a better understanding of Black culture. Finally, and without a clear justification, they also felt that Black physicians would improve research in medical schools and enhance the administration of medical centers. What the authors failed to discuss was whether relaxed admissions would pull down standards across the board.

For many years, physicians have consistently polled among the top two or three most respected professions. Part of this respect derives from the trust the public has in the physician's knowledge and skill. The COVID-19 pandemic again reminded the American people of the need for a highly trained physician workforce that, at crunch time, could implement complex intensive care. Of course, to maintain a highly competent physician workforce requires recruiting the best and brightest students.

Fortunately, there have always been many more applicants than openings for entry into medical school. In recent years, there have been almost two would-be doctors for every available place into both allopathic medical schools and osteopathic schools. Given the numbers, medical schools have great discretion in constructing their first-year classes. As serious as the responsibilities of a doctor are, it would seem logical for schools to recruit the most talented students.

Unfortunately, that is not how things now work. In the not-too-distant past, however, premed students competed fiercely to be among the elect. Indeed, we were the campus buzzkills. If we wanted to get into a medical school, especially a good one, we had to study and study hard. The criteria for admission were simple: grades in college for science courses, scores on the Medical College Admission Test (MCAT), and an interview assessing ethical standards and communication skills. Those whose family name wasn't inscribed in marble above the medical school doors needed to do well on all three of these criteria. When I took the MCAT in 1965, MCAT measured our verbal ability, quantitative ability, science achievement, and knowledge of "general information."

The MCAT, which was first administered in 1928, was part of a reform movement launched a few years earlier. The original MCAT, as noted by Jules Dienstag, former dean of medical education at Harvard Medical School, was developed as an initiative to allow only qualified students to matriculate. The modern approach to undergraduate medical education, one in which students are exposed to the scientific disciplines underlying modern medical care, was completely foreign to most medical trainees at the beginning of the twentieth century. There was no requirement to attend college prior to medical training. Curricula were not standardized. And there were no licensure exams to guarantee at least minimal competence. Students could acquire a medical degree by simply spending time with a practitioner as a mentor. They rarely had the opportunity to care for patients under the supervision of the medical school faculty.

Johns Hopkins, Harvard, the University of Pennsylvania, and the University of Michigan, to name a few, had already adopted a rigorous European model of medical education. But most medical degrees in the United States were granted either by single practitioners who mentored students or by for-profit schools that had no basic requirements for admission other than the ability to pay for the lectures. Seeing the widespread irregularities, the Carnegie

Foundation commissioned Abraham Flexner, a nonphysician, to evaluate the state of medical education and propose reforms. In 1910, Flexner issued his influential report.

Prior to Flexner's report, most medical school attendees were high school graduates. He proposed that medical schools require all matriculants to be college graduates with at least several science courses under their belts. He also recommended that the preclinical time in medical school be expanded to two years rather than the typical eight months at many unaccredited schools. This was the time for students to learn the basic scientific principles underlying the diagnostic skills and therapies they would learn in the clinical arena. Finally, he proposed that medical schools be closely aligned with a teaching hospital at which clinician-educators could supervise the students in learning clinical medicine. This reform movement, while forcing many medical schools to close, launched the modern era of academic medical education in the United States.

True to form, the authors of the AMA master plan see the Flexner report as a source of shame. As they see it, Flexner had a "devastating impact" on women in medicine and "cemented in place" separate but unequal medical training for African Americans. As shall be seen, some activist physicians today have launched a "Beyond Flexner" movement. It does not bode well for medical education.

Flexner helped standardize medical training, but admissions criteria remained flexible. Many medical schools openly discriminated against Blacks, Jews, Italians, and Irish. Most, however, did it subtly through the quiet use of quotas. The most pervasive discrimination during the years 1920 to 1950 was against Jews, and the Ivy League was arguably the chief offender. To a large degree, Jews were able to circumvent these practices, thanks in part to the then New York State Gov. Thomas Dewey, who opened four publicly supported nondiscriminatory universities. Although private, NYU absorbed many Jewish medical students, including the future Dr. Jonas Salk, who had been rejected elsewhere.

Discrimination against would-be Black doctors was not as systematic as it was against Jews, but it certainly existed, and where it did, the doors were firmly shut. Well into the twentieth century, most Black physicians graduated from either Howard University College of Medicine in Washington or the Meharry Medical College in Nashville, both of which opened in the years after the Civil War and both of which passed muster with Flexner.

By the time I entered medical school in 1965, state and federal laws effectively ended systemic racism in medical school admissions. As it happens, that was the same year the Lyndon Johnson administration launched the era of affirmative action, not with a constitutional amendment or even the passage of a bill through Congress, but rather with an executive order. Some medical schools adopted affirmative action programs of their own, as Allan Bakke learned the hard way when he famously applied to the University of California, Davis, in 1973.

In the 1978 case, *Regents of the University of California v. Bakke*, a deeply divided Supreme Court allowed for the continuation of affirmative action to remedy past injustices and only then if there were a "compelling interest" to do so. In his essay, Cohen conceded that certain laws and court rulings have interfered with the advance of the affirmative action agenda, but he showed no great respect for those laws or sympathy with those like Bakke—a thirtysomething military vet—the laws were designed to protect.

Nearly forty-five years after Bakke, as those historic injustices fade further from view, affirmative action is more aggressive than ever. The inarguable reality is that Blacks are preferentially admitted to medical school. Once admitted, they are virtually guaranteed to graduate. And once graduated, they are likely to find training programs more than eager to accept them in the name of diversity.

The attrition rate for students entering medical school sixty years ago was an average of 9 percent although at some schools it was as high as 14 percent.[8] Poor academic performance was

---
8. D. G. Johnson, "The AAMC study of medical student attrition: overview and major findings," *Journal of Medical Education* 40, no. 10 (October 1965): 913–20, https://www.aamc.org/media/15316/download.

the primary reason students dropped out prematurely. Students who left because of nonacademic issues tended to have lower than average grades but were not failing academically. Many returned to school at some point and eventually graduated.

By the 1990s, the medical student attrition rate had declined slightly but was still as much as 5 percent in some academic programs. By 2019, however, the reported attrition rate from medical school was less than 3 percent. This contrasts with law school, where the attrition rate averages 11 percent, or nursing school, where it approaches 20 percent. Ironically, medical educators view the current low rate as an important advance for medical education. In their minds, it signals a more nurturing and supportive environment. Perhaps that is true, but the low attrition rate raises a real concern.

Assuming that students today are no more intelligent or diligent than they were in the 1960s, the decrease in attrition from 9 percent in the early 1960s to 3 percent in 2019 suggests a lowering of standards. Indeed, if the 1960's standards had been applied to the current cohort of students, nearly 800 physicians entering the health-care workforce each year would have failed out of medical school.

Some questions need to be asked about the low dropout rate. Are administrators better at selecting applicants despite no major change in the percentage of applicants accepted? Are students better prepared at college to succeed in medical school? Or are lower standards for medical school success the real reason? From my experience, I'd say "C"—lower standards. Not only has there been a decline in the standards used for admission, but there has also been an ongoing failure to hold students to consistent standards during medical school.

Attrition rates declined when the academic medical community committed to admitting a much higher proportion of underrepresented minority students. It was widely understood that admission standards might be compromised by basing admission on factors other than an applicant's MCAT scores and previous academic performance, but the demand for equity in admissions was powerful. To be clear, "equity" does not mean equality of opportunity. Equity means equality of outcome.

Cohen's plan to enhance Black admissions, at least in terms of numbers, worked out well. According to AAMC data, the number of Black students graduating from medical school in 2000 rose by 50 percent by 2020. This increase was mostly driven by a change in accreditation requirements introduced by the Liaison Committee on Medical Education (LCME), the medical school accrediting body. Medical schools were now required to describe their plans for recruiting more minority students or risk being denied full accreditation.

Much of the enhanced recruiting came at the expense of historically Black colleges and universities (HBCU). In the year 2000, before the new accreditation requirements, nearly one-third of Black medical school graduates came from the medical schools associated with HBCUs. By 2020, the percentage had fallen to less than 10 percent. Despite an acceptance rate of more than 40 percent for all Black applicants, African Americans represented only 8.4 percent of medical students in 2019, considerably less than their 13 or so percent in the population writ large.

Here's the reality: Admitting more minority students compromised admission standards. A study by the American Enterprise Institute using AAMC data in 2017 showed the impact of the diversity initiative on objective measures of academic standards. Black students with a middling GPA in college and a 50ish percentile rank on the MCAT had a ninefold greater chance of admission than Asian students and a sevenfold greater chance than White students. In other words, while only 20 percent of White applicants with such mediocre grades and scores were admitted to a medical school, 85 percent of comparable Black applicants were.

The 2020–2021 data published by the AAMC confirms just how heavily weighted the admission process is. While the four-part MCAT exam is not a requirement for accreditation, most medical schools use it as a measure of a student's suitability for admission. The MCAT, for instance, has a range of only 56 points, 472 to 528. The mean is 500. The average Black applicant scored below average at 498. The average Hispanic—and I am not sure I know why Hispanic is a separate category—scored 501. The average White scored 508, and the average Asian 509. Of interest, Black and Hispanic applicants made up no lost ground on the "Psychological, Social, and Biological Foundations of Behavior" section of the test.

The science GPA numbers are equally telling. For Black applicants, it was 3.17, for Hispanics 3.32, for Asians 3.53, and for Whites 3.57. Despite the better performance by Whites and Asians in both the MCAT and the science GPA, Hispanics were admitted to med school at a higher rate than either Whites or Asians, while Blacks lagged only slightly behind the three other groups: respectively, 40 percent for Blacks, 43 percent for Whites, 43 percent for Asians, and 46 percent for Hispanics.[9] By any reasonable measure, Asians would seem to be more of a "minority group" than Hispanics, but they do not qualify as "underrepresented," which means they don't count as minorities.

Every year and in each of the four phases of the MCAT test, including "Psychological, Social, and Biological Foundations of Behavior," male applicants outscore females. Males also have higher science GPAs. The gap is consistently the most pronounced in the "Chemical and Physical Foundations of Biological Systems" section of the test.[10] Despite consistently better MCAT scores and science GPAs, men and women are being accepted to allopathic medical schools at the same rate, 42 percent. Osteopathic schools do not supply gender data.[11]

---

9. As reported by Shemassian Academic Consulting, https://www.shemmassianconsulting.com/blog/medical-school-acceptance-rates-by-race.
10. Association of American Medical Colleges, "MCAT Scores and GPAs for Applicants to U.S. MD-Granting Medical Schools by Sex, 2018-2019 through 2021-2022," https://www.aamc.org/media/6081/download/.
11. "Medical School Acceptance Rates (2021)," MedEdits Medical Admissions, https://mededits.com/medical-school-admissions/statistics/acceptance-rates/.

As shown in a 2014 study from the University of Kentucky College of Medicine, poor academic performance in college is arguably the best predictor of underperformance in medical school, "underperformance" being defined as having to repeat a course, being placed on academic probation, or suffering dismissal from school. Those matriculants with a lower mean undergraduate GPA were the students most likely to underperform academically in medical school. That only makes sense.

The well-documented grade inflation at US colleges undermines even the GPA as a reliable criterion for admission to medical school. As shown by a study in the carefully researched website, gradeinflation.com, the mean GPA at four-year colleges has been rising at a rate of 0.1 points per decade, and this trend has continued for the past thirty years. The most common grade at a four-year college is now an A. The 42 percent prevalence of A grades inevitably means fewer B and C grades.[12]

While it is possible that students today are performing better than their predecessors, no veteran professor believes this. For the last fifty or so years, student activists have been calling for eliminating grades and adding more "relevant" coursework. Over time, they have had their way. This activism has inevitably led to the weakening of the standards. Then, too, students paying high tuitions are now viewed as "customers" and expect to be treated with deference. They usually are. Administrators cannot afford to lose their tuition money. Finally, faculty members need strong student evaluations for their own career advancement. All of these factors conspire to make grading less rigorous in the vain hope of avoiding student discontent.

In 2004, Princeton University tried to reverse the grade inflation trend. The provost argued that checking grade inflation would reduce student stress by creating uniform expectations. It didn't quite work out that way. The students' failure to secure admission to elite graduate schools, including medical schools, caused an uproar, and the policy was formally rescinded ten years later.

---

12. "Recent GPA Trends Nationwide Four Year Colleges and Universities," https://gradeinflation.com/.

If high grades simply reflect grade inflation, schools should place a greater emphasis on MCAT scores to determine the most appropriate candidates for a medical career. As might be expected, the MCAT too has fallen victim to the social justice censors. A 2008 report from the AAMC advocated for a greater focus on social and behavioral sciences in medical school. Understanding the consequences of bucking an equity trend, MCAT designers went along. Now, 25 percent of the newly formulated exam is devoted to behavioral sciences and the individual's role in society. By undermining hard sciences in favor of social sciences, the medical establishment yielded to the social justice bullies. That faction of medical sociologists who would rather see physicians exploring community social issues than developing cutting-edge care had their way.

In 2012, test designers described the rationale for the changes in the *New England Journal of Medicine*. "Future physicians will need broader skills and knowledge than previous generations," they argued unconvincingly. "It may be as important for aspiring physicians to understand patients' social, environmental, and personal characteristics and complex health care systems as to grasp basic biologic processes."[13] Again and again, the claim that knowing a patient's social characteristics provides insight into his or her disease process is offered without even a passing effort at proof.

We can be assured that correct answers to the questions about social characteristics did not stray far from the current Progressive ideology. That said, the MCAT is still the best means to judge a candidate's qualifications for medical school.

In recent years, the average MCAT score of the first-year med school class has become an important component in the ranking system devised by *U.S. News and World Report*. Why this second-tier magazine has such an impact on administrative self-esteem is a mystery to me. Yet faculty, alumni, trustees, and

---

13. Robert M. Kaplan, Ph.D., Jason M. Satterfield, Ph.D., and Raynard S. Kington, M.D., Ph.D., "Building a Better Physician — The Case for the New MCAT," *New England Journal of Medicine* (April 5, 2012), https://www.ncbi.nlm.nih.gov/pmc/articles/PMC5561547/.

the press pay close attention to each year's assessment. In some cases, the assigned rank even factors into a med school administrator's year-end bonus.

Schools report the MCAT scores along with other data each year. There is one major problem here. As noted, Black students tend to score substantially lower than White or Asian students. Given the imperative to adhere to diversity goals, the MCAT, even watered down, is an obstacle to so-called "equity." As a result, many schools continue to explore ways to justify admitting students without needing to rely on the MCAT, a reliable indicator of their med school success.

To achieve the requisite diversity, many schools have developed "feeder" programs with universities, allowing students to avoid the MCAT exam. These arrangements include combined BA-MD programs in which students spend two years in the undergraduate program and three years in medical school to acquire both degrees. Also, there are direct agreements between colleges and medical schools to admit a certain number of students, typically minority students, if they remain in good academic standing. These programs do not require MCAT scores for admission.

Playing along, *U.S. News & World Report* exempts such programs from MCAT reporting. Currently, fifty-two allopathic and osteopathic medical schools have "pathway programs" that circumvent the reporting of MCAT scores.[14] Given the predictive value of the MCAT exam for success in medical school, only the hopelessly woke believe that waiving the MCAT requirement does *not* erode the integrity of the medical school admission process. Then, too, only an ideologue could believe that the erosion of admission standards does *not* mean future risk to the public.

---
14. Consortium of Accelerated Medical Pathway Programs, https://www.acceleratedmdpathways.org/.

Chapter 5

Dumbing Down

In truth, "diversity" did not have to signify a decline in standards if the curriculum and the assessment of student performance remained rigorous, but it hasn't. The dumbing down begins early, likely in pre-K, but for our argument let's stick to premed.

The premedical curriculum is now being infected by the notion that a rigorous approach to medical education is as obsolete as the ideal of the physician as a highly trained clinical scientist. Traditionally, acceptance into medical school was determined by grades in four or five science courses such as chemistry, physics, biology, organic chemistry, and biochemistry. Unsurprisingly, given the decline in standards for undergraduate medical education, there is a movement afoot to make preparation for medical school less stressful and more, well, friendly.

Recently, Lorenzo Arvanitis, a reporter at the *Yale Daily News*, investigated the state of premedical education from both the students' and medical school faculty's perspectives. As part of his analysis, he describes the plight of Emma, a Yale premedical student overwhelmed by the demands of her science courses:

> In 2017, Emma entered Yale College and noticed many of her peers signing up

for a diverse spread of courses and activities. But her first-year experience was to be much more focused. "I talked to students who were applying to medical school and figured out what I needed to do," she explained. "So, my first year I was taking chemistry, biology and math. I started working in a lab."[15]

Emma's plight troubles reporter Arvanitis. Her story, he realizes, is not uncommon. "From the time they set foot on campus," he gripes, "[premed students] say they must fully dedicate themselves to a rigid lineup of courses and activities that leaves little room for much else." He quotes another premed student who confirms his thesis. His experience in premed, the student assures him, "has definitely taken away from the number of subjects I'm interested in but haven't been able to take."

Arvanitis finds at least one physician who endorses his idea that the connection between the science requirements and the reality of practicing medicine is "blurry and tenuous." Says Dr. Anna Reisman, a 1986 Yale graduate and a professor at Yale's medical school, "Do you really need those classes to be a doctor? Do I refer to my knowledge of any of those subjects in my day to day life when I'm seeing patients? Not really."

Part of the problem here is clearly Dr. Reisman. It is worth examining her background to see why she is so skeptical of hard science. Dr. Reisman is a primary care physician and head of the Yale Program for Humanities in Medicine. To be fair, many primary care physicians are incredibly knowledgeable. They take on the care of the very ill and counsel patients on maintaining healthy lifestyles and treating chronic conditions like diabetes and hypertension.

That said, most primary care physicians are not tasked with treating patients with advanced diseases such as cancer, end-stage

---

15. Lorenzo Arvanitis, "Losing Track," *Yale Daily News*, April 29, 2021, http://features.yaledailynews.com/blog/2021/04/29/losing-track/.

heart failure, end-stage kidney disease, stroke, or any surgical procedures. Dr. Reisman doesn't feel a need to understand the basic science given that a primary care physician is rarely if ever called upon to introduce new treatment modalities. These are first employed by specialists trained in the details of fields such as cardiology, nephrology, endocrinology, and the various surgical subspecialties, among others.

Dr. Reisman likely spends more time counseling patients than treating severe complications. Counseling is valuable but quite a different task than planning a chemotherapy regimen or dealing with the latest cell therapy. Physicians need a strong scientific background to understand the implications of the latest therapies and to employ them most effectively. Having a deep understanding of disease mechanisms and the actions of drugs helps the physician appreciate the individual symptoms that each patient can manifest. That is how the best doctors think.

The story does not end well for Emma with respect to her medical aspirations. Apparently, she found fulfillment working in a bakery, a sign that she was probably not cut out for medicine in the first place. For Mr. Arvanitis, rigorous scientific training only stands in the way of developing the "right" kind of doctors:

> There is no evidence that the cumbersome course load so deeply rooted in the sciences is producing better doctors. Instead, what it seems to be doing is keeping out good people—people from diverse backgrounds who are greatly underrepresented in the profession, people we need as this country sees an ever-growing shortage of primary care doctors. As students like Emma decide to drop the pre-med track, society loses future phenomenal, big-hearted, devoted doctors.

This is yet another example of a profound misunderstanding of the dual roles of a physician—a comforter of the distressed *and* a knowledgeable clinical scientist able to provide the latest therapies to suffering patients. For the last eighty years, American doctors have dominated the Nobel Prize for medicine or physiology. Looking through their résumés, I would venture that every one of them had a strong science background and that each applied that knowledge on a regular basis. Yes, the kindly physicians are important but without hard scientific knowledge and skill, they are often ineffectual.

If these undergrads move on to medical school, most will graduate in four years with more than $200,000 in debt. Some think the expense is worth it. Students will have a degree that guarantees a lifetime income and a large measure of respect in their communities. In reality, a costly medical school education often fails students and risks the future of the medical profession.

Medical school should provide a student with a rich understanding of the basic science that explains the mechanisms of disease and the basis of therapeutic interventions. It should produce young physicians who are prepared for the mastery of their chosen specialties but who are also ready to step into emergency situations and provide needed care for acutely ill patients. If you believe all this is actually happening, you are badly deceived.

Chapter 6

The Color of Care

There is perhaps one issue that could justify the current enthusiasm for increased diversity of the medical workforce, namely if Black communities were medically underserved and Black physicians preferred to practice in those communities. Besides "equity" for its own sake, Dr. Jordan Cohen's call for more Black students in medical school in 1997, described earlier, was based on this presumed dynamic.

The data that has been collected on this issue suggests that this rationale is ungrounded. When Black students or residents are surveyed, they typically indicate their willingness to practice in underserved communities. That much is true. Surveys of physician distribution bear this out: a higher percentage of Black doctors practice in medically underserved areas (MUAs) than Whites. A survey of 48,388 physicians in California confirmed that Black doctors are almost twice as likely to practice in an MUA as White doctors, but White doctors outnumbered Black doctors in that cohort roughly 19:1, 29,797 to 1,555. In real numbers, 4,171 White doctors but only 419 Black doctors were practicing in MUAs.[16]

---

16. Kara Odom Walker, Gerardo Moreno, and Kevin Grumbach, "The association among specialty, race, ethnicity, and practice location among California physicians in diverse specialties," *National Library of Medicine* (Jan–Feb 2012), https://pubmed.ncbi.nlm.nih.gov/22708247/.

Given the relatively small number of Black physicians and the modest interest shown by Blacks in applying to medical school, the pursuit of "equity," even if achieved would have a minimal impact on the MUAs. A 5 percent increase in White commitment to MUAs would have as much effect as doubling the number of Black physicians without any compromise in the quality of the doctors committed to those communities. The sensible answer is to train more good doctors, ignore their skin color, and give them incentives to serve MUAs.

What is not well understood is that the designation of MUA for a community does not necessarily indicate that there is a lack of medical services in the community. The government has decided to define MUAs as follows from the HHS website:

> Medically Underserved Areas/Populations are areas or populations designated by HRSA [Health Resources and Services Administration] as having too few primary care providers, high infant mortality, high poverty or a high elderly population.[17]

It should be noted that Black communities are not necessarily MUAs. In a typical state like Missouri, for instance, the state's two most heavily African American service areas—St. Louis and Kansas City—have an MUA index right in line with the state's more rural counties. Residents of those cities also have much more immediate access to high-level care, especially emergency care, than do residents of outlying areas.

The West Philadelphia neighborhood, the home of the University of Pennsylvania medical center with more than two thousand physicians on staff and a whole hospital of pediatricians, is an MUA according to the government. The problem is obviously not access to medical care; the problem is something else. The high infant mortality rate, high poverty rate, and advanced

---

17.   MUA Find, https://data.hrsa.gov/tools/shortage-area/mua-find.

age of the community are going to persist despite the ethnicity of the physicians in the community. Could moving facilities out of the medical center ten or twenty blocks to the west improve care? Perhaps, but there is minimal if any evidence for that outcome.

Yes, there is abundant medical literature that purports to show that Black patients do better with Black doctors, but this literature deserves some scrutiny. As "exhibit A," consider an article published in 2020 in the *Proceedings of the National Academy of Sciences*. The authors created a sensation among medical practitioners by arguing that Black newborns had a much greater chance of survival if they had a Black neonatologist care for them.

The study mined a large database of newborns in Florida. It compared the outcomes of babies delivered by Black doctors to that of White doctors. To a colleague who was chief of neonatology at a Penn teaching hospital, this whole exercise seemed absurd. Absurd or not, within a few months of publication, fourteen other articles cited this one as further proof, if proof were needed, of medical racism. CNN headlined the results, "Black newborns more likely to die when looked after by White doctors." Science News and Fox News had similar scare headlines.

There is an aphorism in medical research that extraordinary claims require extraordinary evidence. A closer examination of the Florida study undermines its claims. Ethan Milne, a PhD student, wrote a careful assessment of the study for the website, medium.com, and pointed out the study's major methodological weaknesses.

Most were obvious to an informed reader. First, the authors could not identify the race of all the doctors involved in the care of neonates. Second, as is always the case, patient outcomes depended on the team caring for the patient. If an emergency occurred at 3 a.m., it was not the attending physician who cared for the patient. It was the nurses and on-call physicians who ministered care.

Finally, and most importantly, as noted previously, assessing clinical care through database analysis is notoriously wanting. The data sources simply do not provide enough information to judge the true situation. For example, if Black doctors practicing at rural hospitals transferred the sickest or most fragile newborns to large teaching hospitals staffed by predominately White doctors, then the White doctors would likely have a record of higher mortality for their patients simply because the babies were desperately ill when they arrived.

To reach any meaningful conclusion, researchers should have assessed each baby that died by reviewing his or her medical record and determining, to the degree possible, the contribution of the attending physician to the unfortunate outcome. This was not done. Likely, it could not have been done. But without this sort of analysis, the researchers should not have concluded anything save that further study was in order. To suggest that racist White doctors were killing Black neonates was reckless. Yet, the authors, when interviewed, were quick to cite racism as the cause. From an interview conducted by sciencenews.org in August 2020:

> Black doctors may be more in tune with the specific experience that black newborns are facing, [such as] more challenging births as the result of increased socioeconomic pressures.

And

> We also have our physician workforce being trained in a way that is not always fully attentive to the impact of racism, both in the lives of their patients that they are serving or will eventually serve, but also the history of racism within our health care delivery system.

This nonsensical analysis suggests that non-Black physicians who are devoted to caring for premature or ill newborns somehow fail to adequately treat these patients because they are oblivious to the history of the Black experience in the United States. There is no explanation as to how the race of the attending physician, let alone the physician's knowledge of the 1619 Project, somehow produced the disparate outcome. Logic does not matter to these researchers. It is no match for the thrill of imputing racism to others.

A 2018 study published in the *Journal of the American Society of Nephrology* provided a better test of the thesis that Black doctors provide optimum care for Black patients. The study evaluated how frequently Black veterans with chronic kidney disease were referred to specialists to optimize their care. The investigators admitted that they expected to find bias against Black patients. This, in itself, is a much too common state of mind among investigators working in the burgeoning field of "equity science."

The excellent VA electronic medical record allowed the investigators to determine the referral patterns of 56,767 veterans. What they found is that 72 percent of 12,747 Black patients but only 50 percent of 39,767 White patients were referred for specialty care. Despite more expert care, 34 percent of Black patients but 14 percent of White patients unfortunately experienced progression of their kidney disease to a more advanced stage. Clearly, denial of advanced care was not the cause of disparate health outcomes.

Unlike with many diseases and many patient populations, kidney disease and the VA patient population provide robust information on large numbers of patients. I believe this study is more reliable than most observational studies of bias in patient care. It avoids many of the methodologic weaknesses of most such studies.

Many studies suggest that patients are more likely to adhere to treatment plans if they have trust in their physicians. Studies of Black patients and other minority groups conducted at the University of California School of Medicine in 2011 found that many Black patients distrusted the health-care system, particularly if they had had personal experience of what they perceived as discrimination. This distrust was not confined to Black patients. Hispanic and Asian patients expressed similar sentiments.

Distrust and communication problems may contribute to

poor adherence to treatment programs as well as a reluctance to undergo certain tests or procedures. Examples abound of the disparate use of technology and screening tests among Black populations. COVID-19 vaccine hesitance among some African Americans is the most recent manifestation of disparate treatment despite vigorous efforts of the government and the medical community to overcome the resistance.

What is more, there is ample evidence that a racial concordance between patients and physician produces no clinical benefit. In a 2011 study of 22,440 patients over 5 years using a validated government survey instrument, researchers from the University of California Davis School of Medicine concluded, "Greater matching of patients and providers by sex and race/ethnicity is unlikely to mitigate health disparities." There are three other studies that suggest relatively negative outcomes when patients and physicians are matched by race.

In seeking evidence of racism to explain health disparities, some investigators study the dynamics of the interactions between physicians and their Black patients. These studies inevitably suffer from an all too obvious confirmation bias. For example, investigators studying the physician-patient interaction in hypertension cases concluded that racial bias led to suboptimal care for Black patients. This study became a touchstone for other workers in the field. It is cited in more than three hundred medical articles.

Again, however, a careful review shows that the results are considerably less than conclusive. The research team examined the length of time of outpatient encounters and the quality of those interactions between physicians and their patients, Black and White. Using voice recordings and various rating systems, the researchers compared the experience of White patients who had their blood pressure well controlled to that of Black patients whose blood pressure was poorly controlled. They found that Black patients had shorter visits with the physician and a poorer quality of interaction. In sum, they were generally less satisfied with the exchange.

The researchers concluded what they set out to confirm, namely that these physicians were biased against Black patients and that this bias likely contributed to the Black patients' suboptimal blood pressure control. Left unsaid by many of those citing the study was that White patients whose blood pressure was poorly controlled were equally unhappy with their physicians. Likewise, patients whose blood pressure was well controlled, Black or White, had similar experiences. In either case, these experiences were more satisfying than those of the patients whose blood pressure was poorly controlled. Common sense tells us that patients following a successful treatment plan are going to have a more positive interaction with their doctors than those not following such a plan.

Common sense, however, stood in the researchers' way. Of the four possible group comparisons—Black controlled, White controlled, Black poorly controlled, White poorly controlled—they chose to focus on the only one of four possibilities that would show a racial discrepancy, namely White well controlled versus Black poorly controlled. When the demand for evidence of racial bias outstrips the supply, researchers do what they must to meet that demand.

Activists frequently base their claims about systemic bias in health-care workers on data derived from the Implicit Association Test (IAT). The message that racism hunters pull from this test is that doctors have more positive attitudes toward White patients. But the IAT is hardly a gold standard in measuring bias. According to an evaluation by HCD, a consumer marketing company with expertise in psychology, the IAT is less than reliable.

> In psychology, a measure is considered reliable if it has a test-retest reliability of at least 0.7, although it is preferred to be over 0.8. Studies have found that racial bias IAT studies have a test-retest reliability score of only 0.44, while the IAT overall is just around

0.5. The second major concern with IAT is its validity. Validity is best established by showing that results from the test can accurately predict behaviors in real life. However, from 2009 to 2015, four separate meta-analyses came out all suggesting that the IAT is a weak predictor of discriminating behavior.

The IAT measure of bias depends on how quickly a subject responds to pictures of individuals of various races and applies to those pictures descriptive words simultaneously flashed on a screen. If a test subject responds one second more quickly to a picture of a White person with a positive word like "handsome" than to a Black person with the same word that response is said to suggest prejudice. The lack of reproducibility of the test is not surprising, yet many studies in the medical literature rely totally on this assessment.

To label physicians as biased with a highly suspect test like the IAT is slanderous. Researchers need to show actual bias, not present some surrogate assessment. They should also ask themselves a simple question before they even start: What incentives do physicians have to discriminate against Black patients? In my fifty years of medical practice, I have never experienced a physician failing to do all he or she could to care for a Black patient.

Another question: If physicians fail to refer patients to specialists due to bias, what is the gain of not referring them? This supposition is particularly absurd for patients in Medicare. These patients are free to self-refer and are free to visit most physicians. True, they may lack supplemental insurance, so they may have out-of-pocket costs. But that cost is not at the expense of the referring physician. Despite the obvious drawbacks, many of these studies use Medicare databases to assess patient activities.

The same dynamic is true for hospitals. The databases used in studies are almost uniformly created by some insurance entities, and hospitals are reimbursed by those entities. I fail to see any economic rationale for differential treatment based on race for patients in the Medicare system. If there are disparities, it may be because some patients are more inclined to follow through on referrals than others. It is only when a bill to an insurance company or Medicare is generated that follow-through can be documented.

Despite the tens of thousands of man-hours spent on these searches, social justice activists have failed to produce a reliable body of evidence proving that bias or racism explain disparate outcomes of care in any instance. Proof of disparate outcomes is not proof of racism unless we suggest disparate outcomes per se automatically prove "racism." This construct is self-defeating. It will only lead to more distrust of physicians by patients and will undermine efforts to improve behaviors that are the true basis for many relatively poor outcomes.

These clinical examples reveal the problems with applying identity politics to medical care. Diseases must be properly diagnosed before the proper treatments can be applied. Students should be taught the proper diagnostic principles. Only then is therapy possible. Until that body of evidence for widespread racism appears—and it won't—social justice activists should not guide the future of medical education.

Physician activists would serve the community much better by focusing on patients and treating them as individuals rather than envisioning them as hapless members of a victimized cohort. Activists may find it satisfying to speculate on the connection between race and disease or class and disease, but learning about the root causes of poverty or identifying supposed racial discrimination has yet to improve the clinical outcomes for any race or class of patients.

There is a massive need for improvements in living conditions in neighborhoods and communities burdened by poverty, crime, and general decay. These are societal responsibilities and are the domain of politicians, social workers, and voluntary agencies. The idea that physicians have a role in alleviating these social problems will only lead to disappointment all around and less physician availability to practice the craft of healing and counseling.

I am dismayed that so many physicians and so many leaders of the medical establishment accept the premise that the medical system is devoted to harming African Americans. If the system is as rotten as they seem to think, why have the leaders not previously made an industry-wide commitment to send physicians and other health-care workers to antibias training to root out systemic racism? Answer—they have not done so because they know the system is not racist. Nor have they committed themselves to root out the real causes of disparate outcomes such as poverty, poor living conditions, or health illiteracy. In this second case, they have not acted because those are conditions doctors cannot stamp out. Physicians do their best for society when they diagnose and treat patients or find new cures.

I am afraid the embrace of the anti-racist movement by medical leaders is a distressingly cynical maneuver. Its goal is to divert the woke from disrupting a well-functioning enterprise. Administrators everywhere dread the specter of activists savaging them on social media, occupying their offices, even demanding their resignations. They think it shrewder to avoid the pain by confessing to the crime, even if innocent of wrongdoing.

By calling the inequalities between White and Black patients "racism," educators identify a more convenient target than themselves. To further appease their critics, they form committees to study the institution's racist tendencies, remove portraits of dead White men, create newly expanded curricula in social justice, and ensure that every racial quota will be met—no, exceeded—in hiring and admission, Civil Rights Act be damned.

Thanks to these virtuous efforts, institutions can hold out the false promise that the inequalities that minorities are alleged to experience will no longer exist, and the "racists" will be reeducated or, better yet, removed. By the time young trainees realize that despite these efforts, not one more Black patient has escaped a complication of COVID-19, not one more Black woman has escaped a complication in pregnancy, and not one more Black elder has escaped the ravages of diabetes or hypertension, they will all have moved on in their medical careers.

Unfortunately, this virtue signaling will have its costs. The incessant drumbeat—racism, racism, racism—will only further alienate African American patients from their ethnically diverse health-care providers. On the COVID-19 front alone, this message has already reduced the acceptance of critical vaccinations and perpetuated the burden that African American communities have previously experienced.

Medical schools and academic medical societies must be honest with their young trainees and other constituents. Rooting out "racism" in medicine offers little hope of improving medical outcomes for minority communities. The opposite outcome is much more likely. Indeed, there is no messaging more "mixed" than telling vaccine-hesitant African Americans they should trust your "systemically racist" institution and then blaming their failure to heed your advice as another sign of systemic racism.

Penn Medicine, in a manner repeated at virtually every medical school in the United States, has launched a strategic plan to further rid itself of the imagined bane of racism. It has pledged in the education component of its plan to produce a bias-free curriculum, a diverse student body, and graduates prepared to "advance equity." Its overall goal—you guessed it—is to "achieve health equity."

Amid these pillars of the medical establishment, virtue signaling is on full display. For all their piousness, these plans fail to address the real social problems that are the basis for poor health outcomes. And they fail to address the need for communities of color and individuals of color to accept agency for their own health. This means, for starters, adhering to medical treatment and avoiding destructive behaviors.

COVID-19 presents an excellent opportunity to exercise that agency. Leaders in the Black community need to guide individuals to partner with the health-care system, much as Bishop T. D. Jakes has done. "Here's my unsolicited counsel," the *Wall Street Journal* quoted Jakes as saying. "Do your own research. Pray. Consult multiple credible sources, from your personal physician to federal agencies like the CDC. Your earnest quest for truth could save your life—and your loved ones."[18]

---

18. T. D. Jakes, "Prayer and Science Led Me to the Vaccine," *Wall Street Journal*, February 25, 2021, https://www.wsj.com/articles/prayer-and-science-led-me-to-the-vaccine-11614295606.

Chapter 7

Hypercritical Race Theory

A particularly worrisome new tool in the toolbox of medical research is critical race theory (CRT). As seen through the CRT lens, all behavior and all actions are rooted in a racial context. Simply put, every less-than-ideal aspect in the life of a Black citizen can be attributed to racism. Racism, again, is redefined as any discrepancy between the White and Black experience. Nothing bad is attributable to an individual's behavior or choices, let alone to the genetic or cultural characteristics of the group to which that individual belongs. Everything bad is a result of oppressive attitudes or policies ingrained in a society historically dominated by privileged white males. The youthful radicals of White Coats for Black Lives assure us that this is true. "With regards to medicine in particular," they assure us, "risk is conceptualized in a way that shifts blame and responsibility to individuals and 'biological difference' as opposed to the oppressive structures that directly impact individuals and communities."[19] In other words, an individual's genetics and life choices have less impact on his or her health than does that person's place in America's imagined caste system. Stop, *please*. This is malpractice.

---
19. "Our Vision and Values," White Coats for Black Lives, https://whitecoats4blacklives.org/wp-content/uploads/2021/07/WC4BL_Vision_Document_1_.pdf.

In that same spirit, physicians conducting a study at Harvard Medical School and Brigham and Women's Hospital in Boston proudly proclaimed that the study was conducted through the lens of critical race theory. Since this school and this hospital rank at the very top of rating systems for school and hospital excellence, the findings carry great impact.

The physicians, affiliated with Harvard, found that White patients at their institution were more likely to be sent to specialized heart treatment units than Black patients. Black patients, on the other hand, were less likely to be admitted to the specialized units and more likely to be referred to a general medical unit. In follow-up, Black patients were more likely to be readmitted to the hospital within thirty days of discharge from the initial admission.

This readmission disparity, of course, was supposed to suggest inferior care the first time around. The authors were not shy about accusing the referring ER physicians of racism, claiming, "Provider bias against minority patients is pervasive."[20] As always, however, there were other important differences besides skin color.

For instance, proportionately more of the Black patients had coexistent kidney disease and were on dialysis treatments. All patients with kidney disease are at risk for frequent hospital admissions. Dialysis treatments solve the problem of fluid overload, the key problem addressed in this study. Referring patients to a unit in the hospital where such dialysis treatments are best arranged and performed is common practice. In many hospitals, those patients with fluid overload and kidney failure are handled quite differently from those patients with fluid overload due primarily to heart failure. Also, kidney failure patients are frequently readmitted to the hospital for a variety of reasons.

The Harvard researchers engage in pure speculation by attributing the higher thirty-day readmission rate of Black patients to poor care. Kidney failure requiring dialysis treatment alone is a

---

20. Lauren A. Eberly et al., "Identification of Racial Inequities in Access to Specialized Inpatient Heart Failure Care at an Academic Medical Center," *AHA Journals* (October 29, 2019), https://www.ahajournals.org/doi/full/10.1161/CIRCHEARTFAILURE.119.006214.

key factor in determining further in-hospital treatment and even site of care. By assuming the validity of critical race theory, the authors of the study found what they wanted to find rather than a more prosaic cause for the different treatment patterns.

On average, too, many more of the White patients studied had valvular heart disease than did the Black patients. Black patients with valvular heart disease would also have been referred to specialized cardiac units, but proportionately, there were simply fewer of them. Again, the disparity has nothing to do with race.

As is normative in these kinds of studies, the authors never bothered to query the ER physicians about their seemingly different handling of the two populations. If they had done so, the explanations from the ER doctors might have undermined the authors' biased conclusion about their own colleagues' treatment decisions. The investigators could have noted this qualifier in the discussion of their findings, but again, that would have weakened the case for systemic racism.

This study did produce one thing of note, namely the most infamous recommendation of any medical study in the past several years. Badly misinterpreting their own findings, the physician-authors opted to create a system of medical apartheid. Their prose is rough, but their meaning is clear.

> Sensitive to these injustices, we have taken redress in our particular initiative to mean providing precisely what was denied for at least a decade: a preferential admission option for Black and Latinx heart failure patients to our specialty cardiology service. The Healing ARC will include a flag in our electronic medical record and admissions system suggesting that providers admit Black and Latinx heart failure patients to cardiology, rather than rely on provider discretion or patient self-advocacy to

determine whether they should go to cardiology or general medicine. We will be analyzing the approach closely for the first year to see how well it works in generating equitable admissions. If it does, there will be good reason to continue the practice as a proven implementation measure to achieve equity.[21]

Rather than relying on good medical practice, rather than referring patients to the most appropriate site of care, the authors will now base their admission decisions on the patient's skin color or, in the case of "Latinx," their ethnicity. This is probably illegal but certainly immoral and an abrogation of the authors' medical oath to care for the best interests of the patient. That Harvard allows this is shameful. Said a typically spineless hospital spokesman, "The Brigham is committed to examining and eliminating the many impacts that racism has on the health and well-being of our patients."[22] Sure, swell.

Manhattan Institute fellow Chris Rufo, who has been leading the charge against critical race theory, had a different opinion, a much more defendable one. "Now medical professionals are setting the conceptual framework to deny medical treatment to Whites in order to achieve 'non-disparate' outcomes," said Rufo. "This is a moral crime, a violation of the 14th Amendment, and a direct contravention of their oath to 'do no harm.'"

The high infant and maternal mortality rate of Black women are frequently cited as still another "proof" of racism in medical care. "Black women in our country are facing a maternal health crisis," Vice President Kamala Harris assured us in July 2021, and she knew the "primary reason" why—"systemic racial inequities and implicit bias."[23]

---

21. Ibid.
22. Andrew Mark Miller, "Boston hospital set to offer 'preferential care based on race,'" *Washington Examiner*, April 8, 2021, https://www.washingtonexaminer.com/news/boston-hospital-set-to-offer-preferential-care-based-on-race.
23. Alisha Haridasani Gupta, "The White House issues its first-ever proclamation on Black maternal health," *The New York Times*, April 13, 2021, https://www.nytimes.com/2021/04/13/us/politics/black-maternal-health-kamala-harris.html.

Not satisfied with simple racism in the here and now as an explanation, some have attributed this disparity in outcome to obstetrical practices in the antebellum South. I wish I were kidding. In the journal *Public Health*, Drs. Owens and Fett, neither a medical doctor, argued, "The deep roots of these patterns of disparity in maternal and infant health lie with the commodification of enslaved Black women's childbearing and physicians' investment in serving the interests of slaveowners."

Historical inequities from more than one hundred and fifty years ago are now linked to current outcome disparities as if one must cause the other. Theorists of race have justified this conceit by proposing that detrimental social conditions are responsible for any and all counterproductive behaviors, even if they have to go back two centuries to identify those conditions.

Assessing maternal mortality risk in Black women is a clear example of this approach. Despite Kamala Harris's presumptions about medical racism, the reasons for the increased mortality in Black women are rooted in a wide range of variables, including genetics, poverty, health literacy, and nurse staffing at maternity hospitals. Certain behavioral realities contribute to the problem. Black women tend to become pregnant when they are younger than White women. They tend to have more underlying "comorbid" conditions such as obesity, diabetes, and hypertension. They tend to not seek prenatal care as often as White women despite government programs to support such visits. Each of these factors is associated with increased complications of pregnancy unrelated to skin color.

We could call these differences "systemic racism," but that suggests no racist intent on the part of individuals. Were obstetricians to take classes in unconscious bias every year of medical school, their attendance would not do a thing to alter the factors that contribute to the greater risks of childbirth in the Black community.

Some data suggest the hospitals where Black women tend to seek maternal/fetal care may not have the staff expertise needed to handle more complex pregnancies. The lack of such facilities in poor neighborhoods may be a factor, but better clinical training for physicians would improve outcomes much more than any sensitivity class, and the time spent in such classes is time not spent on producing better clinicians.

Chapter 8

Not So Great Expectations

By the mid-twentieth century, Abraham Flexner's proposals had become accepted practice everywhere. Medical school education created the foundation for a knowledgeable and competent medical workforce. At that time, medical school curricula in the United States consisted of two preclinical years and two years of progressively more substantive clinical experiences. Success in medical school was measured in class rank. Every exam was graded, and every clinical rotation was assessed and graded.

When the time came for students to apply for postgraduate residency positions, class rank and score on the first part of the three-part licensure exam were the main criteria examined by residency programs. In the past, letters of recommendation (formally called "Medical Student Performance Evaluation"—MSPE) were valued.

Students had to pass a series of three examinations before obtaining a medical license. The first was given after the second year of medical school and the second after the third year of medical school. A national standard for medical licensure required that students complete at least one year of postgraduate training, and students took the final exam during the first postgraduate year. Some states imposed added requirements such as personal interviews.

The first two years of medical school consisted of courses providing students with a broad and deep introduction to the medical sciences. The first year typically consisted of courses in the normal structure and function of the human body. Students learned the gross and then the microscopic anatomy of normal organ systems. Biochemistry, genetics, molecular biology, and physiology were all subjects for courses spread over several months.

In the second year, students used the information gained in the first year to learn the structural, functional, and biochemical basis of diseases of the various principal organs of the body. Toward the end of the second year, students were introduced to methods of eliciting a patient's history of their illnesses and to the techniques of the physical examination. Laboratory testing, radiologic techniques, and other ancillary aspects of medical care were introduced at that time as well.

With this strong science background, students were then introduced to clinical medicine by rotating through various hospital or outpatient clinical activities as a member of a clinical team typically made up of senior faculty members and more advanced trainees in residency programs. Experiences in medicine, primary care, surgery, pediatrics, obstetrics and gynecology, emergency medicine, and psychiatry typically comprised the third year of medical school.

In the fourth year of medical school, students began to function as interns in their chosen specialties. They had these more advanced clinical experiences in fields that particularly interested them and in fields related to their chosen specialties. For example, a student interested in surgery might spend time in the department of anesthesia learning the techniques of preparing patients for surgical procedures. Students interested in internal medicine might spend time caring for cardiology patients or patients with gastrointestinal disorders. While these advanced experiences provided the students with increasing levels of responsibility in caring for patients, they were still closely monitored by faculty and advanced trainees. By the time students completed the fourth year, they were ready to be effective participants, for instance, in the clinical care the COVID-19 epidemic demanded.

During these preclinical and clinical experiences, students learned communication skills and the professional aspects of medicine. While these issues were not nearly as prominent in medical school curricula as is the current practice, they were adequately addressed, usually through courses offered by the psychiatry faculty with a focus on communication skills. Students learned professionalism by observing clinician teachers and other senior physicians.

Today's medical school curriculum puts far greater emphasis on communication skills, social topics, and, more recently, the role of systemic racism in medical outcomes. The science content of student education has been dramatically reduced. So has the range of clinical experience. Today, there is a reduced expectation that students immerse themselves in clinical activities during the fourth year of school. These developments, along with a decline in faculty expectations, have diminished the practical value of medical education.

Assessment in medical student performance has become much less rigorous than in previous eras, and that has likely led to less qualified students graduating into the medical workforce. How could it not? The new approach to achieving equity in outcomes has not only allowed the unqualified to progress through the system but has also decreased the motivation for qualified students to gain higher levels of achievement. This has occurred by minimizing competition among students.

Unfortunately, grades are becoming a historic relic, further obscuring the relative merit of medical school graduates and removing one of the strongest motivations for student achievement. Most schools continued to use some grading system for clinical work, but many schools have inflated grades in the clinical courses. In the top-ranked medical schools, some 50 percent of students achieved "honors" in their key clinical courses. In some schools, 90 percent of the students received the highest grade given.

How did this happen? First, educators in medical schools have created extensive curricula in social topics. There are only so many hours in the day for educating students, a reality underscored when social issues occupy a substantial amount of curricular time. In my medical school, a four-year module of the curriculum is called "Doctoring." The module consumes one to three hours of class time per week in the first two years and four to six hours of formal instruction at less frequent intervals in the subsequent years. The curriculum includes readings and lectures on cultural differences in perception of disease as well as many sessions on bias against various groups, most notably the Black and Asian communities.

This is a modest amount of time compared to other schools. For example, in a study carried out by Harvard Medical School, it was found that one out of every four medical schools offers coursework in prison medicine. More dramatic still is the programming at the Geisel School of Medicine at Dartmouth College. Named for Dr. Seuss creator Theodor Geisel (not himself a medical doctor), the school condemns its students to a four-year-long march through the minefields of woke medicine:

> The social justice curriculum there, as published in the medical education literature, includes a minimum of 55 hours of content divided into 30 hours of classroom work (didactic and small group) and at least 25 hours of experiential learning. The 30 classroom hours comprise 15 hours of new large- and small-group teaching, and 15 hours of social justice topics integrated into closely related subjects already addressed in the formal medical school curriculum. The 25 hours

of experiential learning are configured as a mandatory, longitudinal, mentored experience spread over four years and potentially encompassing myriad activities, including volunteerism, community outreach, and scholarly research relevant to social justice.

The phrase "mandatory, longitudinal, mentored experience" sounds like the kind of joyride one might be yoked to in Orwell's Oceania. However progressive these administrators might be, they chose not to scrub Geisel's name off the medical school after it was discovered, in the words of a school official, that "some of his work perpetuated offensive stereotypes." What is scary is that they actually thought about it. "We continue to explore opportunities to contextualize and educate from this chapter of the Geisel legacy," apologized the official in predictably obtuse educational jargon.

These eighty hours at Dartmouth are said to prepare students to solve the disparities in health outcomes among African Americans and other communities. How is this to be accomplished? Who knows? As with all such claims that the social justice curricula will benefit patients, no one ever presents any credible evidence as to how. Educators satisfy themselves with a series of trendy clichés. Here is what the Dartmouth faculty pretend will result from their social justice curriculum as published in the journal *Academic Medicine*:

- Means of addressing health disparities
- The concept of service
- Solidarity with the underserved
- Physician as advocate
- Working as part of a team
- Meeting immediate medical needs

- Community development model
- Building infrastructure
- Skills transfer for sustainability
- Formation of community coalitions
- Trust and listening
- Leadership training
- Conducting community assessments
- How to assess health intervention outcomes
- How to prioritize health interventions
- Comparative healthcare systems
- Service organization business models
- Introduction to medical anthropology
- Cultural and spiritual sensitivity

This miscellaneous apples and oranges list is flat-out embarrassing. How any of this will "address disparities" is not specified because the whole enterprise is ridiculous. The goal of these "outcomes" is clearly political, not medical. The only conclusion that can be reached from reading through this list is that a physician has no more ability to alter health outcomes than does a social worker. Social workers, at least, receive two years of full-time training to learn this stuff. It does not distract from their mission. It is their mission.

The idea that physicians have the time or expertise to carry out the tasks of social workers defies reality. Moreover, the curriculum proposes that physicians will carry out these tasks *gratis*. There is absolutely no discussion in any of these social justice curricula regarding how the time physicians are expected to spend on social issues will be compensated.

One must ask why—when confronted with an aging population, an astonishing growth in biomedical knowledge, and the emergence of new pandemic risks—the medical establishment devotes increasing time to topics that have little if anything to do with healing the sick? The only possible conclusion is that the politics of social justice has so infected the world of medicine that medical educators have become divorced from reality.

The curriculum on social justice assumes that one can be taught how to deal with suffering patients by learning scripts and buzzwords. Most of the teaching sessions in the social justice curriculum seek to inform students of the trials and tribulations of patients living in poverty. But the whole point of a liberal education is to produce students who, through their reading of literature and history, are familiar with the range of human emotions. Shame, doubt, and suffering are universal phenomena.

Can sessions in which students are asked to pretend to give bad news to actors portraying patients really prepare them to tell a family that their child has a brain tumor? Will these sessions teach students how to utter the words that provide the hope and reassurance required? Traditionally, students learned these skills through observing senior clinicians deal with patient suffering in real clinical settings. While a lecture or two may help to set the tone needed for proper interactions with suffering patients, the repetitive sessions during the fifty-five hours of the Dartmouth social justice curriculum offer little besides guilt, division, and unearned pride. In Dartmouth, as elsewhere, medical schools fail to prepare their students for the lifetime of learning and practicing medicine that lies in front of them.

Unfortunately, many medical educators seem to believe that these social diversions are more important than the historic core of medical education—learning the basic science underpinning contemporary medical care. They see physicians playing a major role in organizing health care in communities and being advocates for all sorts of progressive goals.

For too many would-be doctors, medical school has become a credential-generating mechanism that allows a virtue-signaling entry into the social justice arena. They enter not as mere doctors but as warriors. Exploiting the historic prestige of the medical profession, these doctor-activists are well positioned to indoctrinate more adherents to their views. The recent emphasis on "anti-racism" themes in medical education will only serve to encourage their activist instincts at the expense of their medical training. In the way of example, consider this plea in the journal of *Academic Medicine* offered in 2020 by medical educators at Tufts University School of Medicine.

> Physicians in the United States receive little or no training on structural racism during their medical careers and are unprepared to work constructively with racially diverse communities, either individually as clinicians or collectively through advocacy, to address the health problems caused or worsened by racism. In response, scholars developed an anti-oppression curriculum in post-medical training for health professionals to mitigate health care disparities and address provider biases.

This collection of unfounded suppositions reads as naturally as a state-sanctioned op-ed in the Beijing *People's Daily*. It gets worse. The educators continue:

> Such efforts need to occur earlier and more broadly. Students must learn about structural racism, including its historical and continuing manifestations through power, privilege, and policy, and the social epidemiology that links it to health outcomes. Racism is deeply embedded in all aspects of U.S.

society. Physicians need to understand this in order to form more trusting relationships with patients and avoid victim blaming by acknowledging and addressing structural racism during the patient visit.

For the authors, continually repeating jargon about "structural" this and "deeply embedded" that takes the place of offering evidence of actual racism, let alone its effect on medical care. The authors stress in the same article that learning about anti-racism is as important as learning about any other aspect of the medical school curriculum.

But the educators seem to have missed a key point: African Americans come to the hospital for medical care, not liberal condescension. I suspect that Black patients would be as shocked as patients anywhere to learn how much of their doctor's training has been squandered on problems that they are in no position to address.

Progressives have sought to transform medicine from its traditional aim of caring for the sick into a mechanism for curing societal ills. They see as their mission recruiting armies of white-coated soldiers in the war on poverty, poor housing, gun violence, pronoun misuse, and other such real or imagined problems. Students who enter leftist-run institutions—now including virtually all medical schools—quickly learn that service in the woke army is not exactly voluntary.

In 2009, writing in the journal *Academic Medicine*, medical educators at the University of California, San Francisco (UCSF), the fourth-ranked medical school in the United States, investigated how well their students were prepared for further training as residents. As part of the educators' project, they surveyed the directors of the residency programs that trained UCSF medical school graduates on the grads' medical knowledge and general competence.

Given that students who matriculate at an elite medical school like UCSF are among the strongest in the country, one would expect residency program directors to judge them favorably. Alas, not so. The program directors found a full third of the UCSF graduates deficient in basic medical knowledge when they began their first year of residency.[24]

The UCSF study has not been repeated in the past dozen or so years. Since then, med school curricula have only grown less rigorous, thanks to the increased time spent on various social justice topics, the introduction of anti-racist training, and the decline in the standards to which students are held.

Just as many colleges are forced to provide remedial learning plans for recent high school graduates, residency programs, even at the most prestigious institutions, must now do the same. Too many medical school graduates start their residency programs needing remediation in the most basic clinical skills. Will they ever catch up with their peers? They may be soldiers in social justice warfare, but it is unlikely they will be top-notch clinicians.

This is not just an American problem. Many studies of medical student preparation have been conducted in the United Kingdom. Medical education there closely aligns with the American model, as do faculty worries about student preparation. In one study conducted in a teaching hospital at the University of Nottingham, supervising physicians found their first-year residents to be unready for practice, deficient in clinical and practical skills, and even lacking in basic communication skills.

The response of recent medical school graduates to the COVID-19 epidemic illustrates the problem. A new disease arrived, and despite the valiant and even courageous response by frontline physicians, it soon became apparent that the medical workforce was unprepared to care for a large influx of desperately ill patients. This lack of readiness had two explanations. On one hand, there was a shortage of experienced and skilled intensive-care specialists who could treat desperately ill patients.

---

24. Lyss-Lerman et al., "What Training Is Needed in the Fourth Year of Medical School? Views of Residency Program Directors," *Academic Medicine* (July 2009), https://journals.lww.com/academicmedicine/Fulltext/2009/07000/Preparing_Graduates_for_the_First_Year_of.7.aspx.

This was a long-standing issue. Even pre-pandemic, the Society of Critical Care Medicine was warning that only 50 percent of US hospitals had a board-certified intensivist on their staffs.

In 2020, the health-care system needed an all-hands-on-deck approach to take care of critically ill patients. In some locales, such as New York City, these patients began to overwhelm hospital capacity. In a survey of more than five thousand members of the Society of Critical Care Medicine, nearly two-thirds of the physicians and nurses surveyed believed that their ICU team was inadequately prepared to treat COVID-19 patients. Many hospitals called for volunteer physicians to man medicine's front lines for these patients requiring intensive care. Emergency room physicians, cardiologists, surgeons, pulmonologists, and others who were familiar with intensive-care medicine rose to the challenge and performed in ways that could only be called heroic.

On the other hand, many physicians felt completely unable to handle these critically ill individuals. Some could not function as frontline physicians during this epidemic. It is understandable that those older physicians who had practiced medicine for many years in specialties that rarely encountered such ill patients were unable to handle frontline roles. What was worrisome was that many recent medical school grads proved incapable of caring for desperately ill patients.

As an April 2020 *Wall Street Journal* article reported, these young physicians felt overwhelmed. Among the physicians highlighted by a team of four reporters was Rita Morales, a resident at NewYork-Presbyterian Columbia in training to be a psychiatrist. For many days, she and her co-residents counseled patients and managed their medications. When COVID-19 patients started to arrive in numbers, administrators told the psychiatry residents they needed them to help care for the sickest of patients in the intensive-care unit.

"My initial reaction was shock and kind of thinking I can't do this," Dr. Morales told the *Journal* reporters. Upon volunteering to go to the ICU, she found herself in over her head. "I was immediately put to go manage a ventilator." She did not know how. A staffer had to show her.

"In hospitals overwhelmed by Covid-19," reported the *Journal*, "medical residents—young doctors in training for a specialty—are being thrust into roles they aren't prepared for." In this article, the *Journal* reporters seemed unaware that they were reporting on a problem not caused by COVID-19, but exposed by it:

> Working long shifts in overflowing ICUs where supervising doctors are stretched thin, young trainees sometimes watch YouTube videos at home late at night to learn procedures they were never taught. Residents are finding themselves navigating critical decisions alone, in a role they say has left them unable to give patients the level of care and attention they need.
>
> At one hospital, residents said they were told to learn respiratory therapy, a licensed job that requires at least two years of training, from a Zoom session and a Google document.
>
> At another hospital, a patient died on a ventilator with a setting turned too high by residents who didn't know how to operate the device, according to residents there.
>
> A resident at a third institution, just learning to manage a ventilator, described being afraid that patients were being treated as guinea pigs.

To be fair, a generation ago, COVID-19 would have put a strain on any hospital staff. From experience, however, I can assure the reader that the physicians then would have been better able to handle the stress. This past year in my institution, by contrast, few primary care physicians were comfortable treating patients hospitalized with COVID-19. One senior primary care physician told me that he was the only primary care physician to volunteer to treat seriously ill COVID-19 patients. More than seventy-five primary care physicians felt unqualified to do so.

The epidemic also revealed the futility of teaching social justice in medical school. One truth had to shake the confidence of even the most combative of social justice warriors. The *social* ills that made certain people more susceptible to contracting COVID-19 were well beyond any possible physician intervention. Treating the patients' *medical* ills would have been much been more useful and should have been within a physician's skill set. In too many cases, however, physicians lacked the basic know-how. All the time young doctors spent on the so-called "social determinants of health" would have been much more beneficial to the Black community had they devoted that time to learning how to manage patients with very low oxygen levels in their blood.

In this brave new world, circular logic prevails. Many of these students will convince themselves that since they completed the course of study and became physicians, they deserved to be admitted in the first place. Their educators will assure them that they are right. Only the public remains in the dark.

These themes are all part of the Progressive mindset that now dominates medical education and the entire health-care community. To be sure, they have dominated academia for years, but no one dies when an English graduate can't identify *Hamlet* or a history grad confuses the two World Wars. By contrast, people will die when med school grads know less about anatomy or biochemistry than they do—or think they do—about climate change and racial injustice. Without a course correction, medical care in the United States, long admired as among the best in the world, will undergo a slow and painful decline.

Chapter 9

What Price Atonement

The cost of medical education is onerous, some $50,000 to $70,000 per year. The inevitable result is massive debt. In no small measure, the soaring tuition reflects the cost of converting medical schools into indoctrination camps for woke ideology. The tuition also reflects the cost of creating and sustaining a mechanism that assures even the weakest students will graduate. Debt aside, the flow of money through academic medical centers keeps everyone content. The money satisfies the students' ideological demands and buffers their passage to graduation, and it enhances the power, prestige, and paychecks of the educators.

In 2019, Dr. Larry Jameson, the dean of Penn's medical school, was paid more than $3 million in total compensation. Department chair salaries at Penn are not publicly disclosed, but many earn more than $1 million per year. These salaries do not reflect compensation for leading a medical school, but rather, they represent compensation for leading a huge health-care business. Penn Medicine, for instance, has annual revenues of more than $6 billion. It's big business delivering high-end medical services to well-insured patients in six hospitals with more than three thousand staff physicians and tens of thousands of employees.

In most academic medical centers, the medical school faculty belongs to one physician group. The doctors in that group practice exclusively at the affiliated hospital. In return for that service, the hospital subsidizes the academic activities of the medical school. In addition to hospital funding, schools generate research funds, most notably from grants and contracts with the National Institutes of Health (NIH). Schools also generate tuition dollars. It is tuition, of course, that causes the huge debt burden borne by medical students.

At public institutions, the average cost for a four-year med school education is north of $250,000. At private institutions, the cost is just south of $350,000. And that does not include room and board. Why so expensive? Good question. The actual education students receive is not what is driving up the cost. Unlike their peers in liberal arts, med school faculty members receive ample outside income either from practicing medicine or doing research. The institution does not need to pay a full salary for the faculty's teaching efforts.

Also, once students progress into the clinical portion of the curriculum, teaching occurs simultaneously with patient care. This practice increases the time required to care for a given patient, but the incremental time is modest. In these instances, the teaching typically emerges as a conversation between faculty and students. A small number of faculty members function as course directors or teaching supervisors and commit substantial time to education. In the preclinical portion of the curriculum, some faculty members devote as much as half of their work time to education as lecturers or small group preceptors, but this activity rarely lasts more than a week or two for the entire academic year. Course directors in the preclinical year may devote a month or six weeks to their courses. Typically, fund transfers between the hospital and the medical school cover the teaching salaries.

As at all academic institutions, "administration" consumes large chunks of revenue, and those chunks are getting larger by the year.

At Penn, there are eight deans responsible for the medical curriculum and student affairs. They are kept company by more than forty staffers. Staff salaries average about $75,000 per year, and faculty salaries run about $250,000 per person. As costly as this may seem, the overall revenue from tuitions—approximately $40 million per year—well exceeds the cost of running the medical school.

True, many students receive financial aid, but those aid dollars come from monies donated to special tuition funds or drawn from endowments. For better or worse, the way this model works is that schools charge high tuitions, withdraw monies from scholarship funds or educational endowments, and then forward these dollars to the institution's top brass to be used as the brass sees fit.

Universities need to have such unrestricted funds to develop new programs but also to support the very high costs of school administration. For example, Penn garnered more than $750 million in research grants from the federal government, but the budgets associated with that support restrict that money to specific research programs. Then too, the complex clinic programs in the health-care delivery enterprise have huge fixed costs. The revenues generated by this enterprise have to stay in-house.

These various restrictions make tuition money all that much more attractive. Tuition dollars can be spent just about anywhere. The very availability of this money encourages growth in the administration, and that growth fuels further increases in tuition. In short, the cost of "education" has not caused a tuition spike well above the national consumer price index. The cost of administration—nurtured on tuition money and the allure of unrestricted funds—is the culprit.

The unchecked growth in the cost of administration, spurred on by mandates from the accrediting agencies for new social programming, drives the steady increase in tuition. An additional cost driver is the coaching of students who struggle with whatever scientific learning is still required. Since administrators manage this money, not teachers or trainers, they put their needs first.

This helps account for the explosion in the cost of "managing" equity and inclusivity.

One major cause of tuition inflation is the federal student loan program. Since the federal government subsidizes student loans, administrators know they can raise tuition with minimal resistance. Students receive the loans, pay the tuition, and assume more and more debt as the schools continue to raise costs each year. As they say, in for a penny, in for a pound.

According to the Education Data Initiative, this year's medical school graduates owe an average of more than $200,000 in educational debt, premed included. In 1978, the average medical school debt in the US was a little more than $13,000. If that debt had grown at the rate of inflation, it would be less than $60,000 today. In other words, total student debt increased at a rate *four* times faster than the consumer price index (CPI). If debt continues to outpace the CPI at the present rate, the average medical student debt will exceed $300,000 by 2024.[25]

Given the economic benefit to a university of adding a medical school, it should surprise no one that thirty-five new ones have opened their doors since 2000, and this just in the United States. All are affiliated with a teaching hospital and a university, some loosely, but few have a research faculty. In addition to the fungible revenue flow from tuition, a medical school makes the university more attractive. Entering undergraduates correctly believe that matriculating at a university that includes a medical school will increase their chances of acceptance at that medical school.

Predictably, these new schools skew to the woke. The AMA master plan goads them on, urging administrators to "[c]reate and implement an equity training curriculum and plan for training opportunities inclusive of gender & LGBTQ+ equity, anti-racism, and trauma-informed approaches, at minimum, for staff of AMA, JAMA and Health 2047."[26] If administrators wish to win the

---

25. "Research and Resources to Tackle the Rising Costs of Higher Education," *Education Data Initiative*, https://educationdata.org/.
26. "The AMA's strategic plan to embed racial justice and advance health equity," *AMA*, https://www.ama-assn.org/about/leadership/ama-s-strategic-plan-embed-racial-justice-and-advance-health-equity.

respect of their peers and the approval of accrediting organizations, they must dive headfirst into this now mainstream academic zeitgeist. Among the eight listed "values" of one "new" school, the Kaiser Permanente Bernard J. Tyson School of Medicine in Pasadena, are the following:

— Promoting inclusiveness and diversity in medical education and the health professions

— Achieving health equity for all and the elimination of health disparities wherever they exist

— Advocating for change in medical education, the profession, and the healthcare system

— Developing courageous leaders who challenge the status quo with inquiry and innovation

This med school seems more intent on producing revolutionaries than physicians. A 2020 *Academic Medicine* article by Schuster et al. about that new med school features the following boast: "Our Health System Science department has developed curricular material on such topics as poverty, racism, and gender inequities for both case-based classroom learning and a 2-year service-learning course at federally qualified health centers." Yes, but why?

To jump-start the operation, the school will have a tuition-free period for the first five years. Thereafter, it will join the herd and charge $55,000 per year. These tuition costs do not fairly represent the cost of education. They reflect the extraordinary inflation in administrative costs for higher education throughout academia.

To sustain their high salaries, administrators in medical schools and their parent universities cannot risk any disruptions by students and faculty. Better to appease the woke by adopting the latest progressive mania than to antagonize them by demanding academic rigor. A related feature of these new schools is a focus on "wellness" programs for faculty and students. Pampering entitled employees and students who feel the great "stress" of studying calms the potential disruptors and maintains the current order.

Many commentators declare that the cost of medical education is unsustainable, and they are likely correct. The value of the undergraduate medical education provided in medical schools is not worth what these schools are charging. The end product is neither rigorous nor comprehensive. These deficiencies persist in the postgraduate residency programs in which students receive specific training in medical specialties. In some surgical subspecialties, the residency program may last more than four years. But even at these advanced levels, the programs rarely provide the scientific knowledge that should have been taught in medical school. In the absence of that strong background, practitioners will function more like technicians when what the nation needs are well-rounded clinical scientists who can easily adopt new approaches to medical care as medical research advances.

One other economic factor drives the political and ideological agenda of at least some academic medical centers and medical schools. These institutions, at least the oldest and most influential ones, are urban economic engines. They are often the largest employer in their respective area. Penn is one such powerhouse. As such, the academic medical center must navigate local politics to achieve its economic goals.

Given their not-for-profit status, medical schools, medical centers, and their parent universities are forever working to assure they will not be forced to pay real estate and sundry other taxes imposed on for-profit entities. They also must deal with zoning issues to allow for expansions of their health-care and research activities. This leads to a close medical-political nexus with local officials. Much is at stake. In October 2021, for instance, a Chester County, Pennsylvania judge denied Tower Health's bid to secure property tax exemptions for three of its Pennsylvania hospitals. Tower Health, a not-for-profit health-care system anchored by the highly respected Reading Hospital, sought exemptions for its three hospitals based in Chester County. In the decision to deny tax exemptions, the county judge ruled that operations at the three Tower Health facilities had become too similar to for-profit facilities in that they did not provide ample uncompensated services and worked with too many physicians at for-profit facilities.

The issue, in this case, was not the judge's ruling but the initial—and highly subjective—denial by the Chester County Board of Assessment that the judge upheld. In a "blue" county like Chester, the appearance of seeming "for-profit" did not help Tower Health's case. To prevent such actions by cash-strapped local governments, academic medical centers must court government officials as well as the media. They must provide arguments to justify their avoidance of multi-million-dollar tax bills and avoid actions that would offend liberal sensitivities. In America's urban areas, the top officials are almost always Democrats, many of them very liberal. It would be difficult, particularly in the post-George Floyd era, for the largest employer in a city to present anything but a full-throated endorsement of social justice activism.

No one benefits, however, when educators prostrate themselves on the shrine of anti-racism. This is a distortion of traditional community involvement and, paradoxically, feeds into local distrust of the health-care establishment. For leaders to tell the community that they have been racist for years and only now have come to confront this evil does not win anyone's confidence. Vaccine skeptics take no comfort hearing health-care leaders confess past sins, real or imagined. Why should they accept vaccination recommendations now from people who all but brag about their responsibility for, say, the Tuskegee experiment?

Indeed, African Americans have heard more about that misguided experiment in the last year or two than any time in the eighty years since it was launched. The "anti-racists" make sure they do. It is hard to find a clearer example of that cult's malevolent influence on the people they are alleged to be helping.

How the inflationary spiral of medical education will end is anyone's guess. It clearly cannot continue apace unless schools generate new sources of outside support. Other nations pay for medical education, but they typically require a specific return on their investment. For a physician, this could mean assignment to a specific locale or a given specialty. American physicians, even the woke, would likely chafe under such a regimen.

Some schools like the NYU Grossman School of Medicine have declared that it will no longer require any tuition payments from students and will depend on an endowment as the source of funding. Assuming a 5 percent spending rule for endowments and $40 million a year to cover tuition costs, we're talking about an endowment of at least $800 million.

Not surprisingly, critics on the left have attacked this model as encouraging income inequality. They argue that since physicians are so well compensated, it does not seem fair that they should also receive free education, especially if they have financial resources of their own. Let's face it. There is no satisfying these people.

Another possibility is a series of targeted scholarships provided by wealthy individuals. The racial bean counters would wreak havoc on a program like this if the benefactors chose the "wrong" people. Besides, few schools could attract enough affluent donors to make it work. If present trends continue, future taxpayers will likely be asked to subsidize an outlandishly expensive medical education. Med students will endorse this movement at least until they see just how many and restrictive are the strings when the state owns their future.

Chapter 10

Unhelpful Changes

As shown earlier by the doleful assessment of UCSF graduates confronting patients in their postgraduate residencies, the enormous commitment of time and money in medical education no longer assures young physicians are ready to begin their careers treating the ill. The changes in curriculum design and content have produced a generation of physicians less prepared to provide effective care than the generations that came before them. These new doctors may be more sensitive to cultural nuances, but a suffering patient wants relief, not nuance.

Among other unhelpful changes, contemporary medical school curricula have dramatically devalued the scientific basis of disease. At Penn, the curriculum was revamped in the mid-1990s without a real rationale other than that a new millennium was coming and that meant "change" was necessary. Comparably empty "reforms" were implemented in nearly all medical schools during the last thirty years. The common argument for the changes was that the curriculum model—two years of basic classroom teaching in hard sciences such as genetics, biochemistry, physiology, and biostatistics—was outmoded and did not conform to new theories of adult education. But as will be seen, adult education theory is not appropriate for undergraduate medical education. Nowhere has it proven to be a valid model for teaching medical students. Indeed, the notion that traditional medical education was somehow outmoded was pulled from thin air.

Two major changes took place at Penn. First, the time spent on learning the basic sciences in medical school was dramatically reduced from twenty-four months of such instruction to fourteen months. At the heart of modern medicine is biochemistry. Before the reforms, students took five sessions a week in biochemistry for sixteen weeks. Now, they take three or four sessions each week for eight weeks.

Inevitably, students learn less. Instead of exploring in detail the biochemistry of enzyme reactions, energy control in cells, protein synthesis, the mechanism of mRNA action, lipid metabolism, detoxification pathways, bone metabolism, the energetics of muscle function, and many other topics, students primarily focused on energy metabolism in the body.

The same truncation occurred with anatomy. Second-year students sensed they had been shortchanged only when they rotated onto the general surgery service and realized how much they didn't know. All too often, I heard students openly regret their failure to learn more anatomy as that would have greatly helped them understand the surgical procedures they observed. They were right. A course that went on for an entire year in my own medical school experience was now over in three months. A survey course in anatomy does not offer a deep understanding of key anatomic details, and although everyone suffers as a result, ultimately the patient suffers the most.

Some courses, such as pharmacology and the study of therapeutics, have been eliminated altogether. As an alternative, drug usage was to be reviewed only in later cardiology, gastroenterology, and other organ-based courses. The idea was to integrate material from courses based on disciplines such as biochemistry, anatomy, and genetics and embed them into a course on the heart, the lungs, the GI tract, and the like. As a result, the cardiology course had lectures on drug effects on the heart, the anatomy of the heart, the genetics of heart disease, and more. Students also spent time in small group sessions where clinical scenarios were discussed to illustrate the basic principles presented in the lectures.

This sounds efficient, and it would be workable if the students were given enough time to learn this material. They would also have to be given the responsibility for reading deeply on these topics. But the time constraints mean that the material has been taught superficially. The typical student does not read about the topic in question but depends on lecture notes and diagrams provided in the lecture material. To repeat, there are virtually no reading assignments in the science component of medical school.

Advocates for the integrated model point to the high level of student satisfaction. But students are always "satisfied" when coursework takes less time and exams are relatively easy to pass. Besides, why should those who know very little get to decide what "satisfaction" means in a medical school context? Educators have lowered the level of expectation. With the material compressed and the breadth of learning minimized, they would face revolt if they made the exams hard.

I confronted the vice dean for education at Penn regarding the superficiality of the science teaching and the insufficient time spent in developing a personal database of basic biomedical science knowledge. She simply told me that times had changed. Students, I was informed, could simply log on to the internet and look up what they needed to know if they had not learned it previously.

This was the school's justification for a 40 percent reduction in preclinical science training. A comparable justification was used to scrap in-class learning during the COVID-19 panic. These shortcuts didn't work. They never really do. Even at the med school level, especially at the med school level, students benefit when the training is comprehensive and guided by experts.

Ezekiel Emanuel, the vice provost for international study at Penn, is best known as an architect of Obamacare. An oncologist by training, Emanuel called for a dramatic reduction in the time spent learning the scientific basis of medicine. He targeted his anti-intellectual approach to biochemistry training. His timing wasn't great. New insights into the nature of cancer promptly showed the importance of knowing the biochemistry behind the energy production of cancer cells.

Emanuel had a particular aversion for the Krebs cycle, a key but complex metabolic pathway involved in generating the molecules that provide energy for cell function. He liked to declare that students had no need to learn about it. Emanuel should have known better. Time and again, basic biologic principles have been found to be crucial in creating new clinical approaches. Recent studies revealed that the Krebs cycle is a major regulator of cancer cell growth. Many pharmaceutical companies and academic researchers are developing ways of regulating this pathway to treat malignancies. These researchers all know their biochemistry. A patient waiting for a cancer cure would not care a whit if these researchers all failed "Systemic Racism 101."

This foolishness repeats itself over and over; seemingly minor scientific topics become the basis for major advances in therapies. Depriving students of the background information handicaps their facility with incorporating new treatments into their clinical activities.

The itch to compress the time spent on learning basic science rapidly spread through American medical schools. The compression was very popular with students and educators as well. Teachers everywhere, the med schools included, crave student approval. It is not just about self-esteem. Administrators use student assessment of teachers and coursework as key metrics in measuring the quality of student education.

At Penn and elsewhere, the assessment process has become much too dependent on student surveys. Students get to grade teachers on the value those students claim to pull from lectures and small group sessions. Those grades become a crucial part of the teacher's dossier for promotion. A professor who challenges the student with difficult material or whose course examination is perceived as too difficult risks a student backlash. Not wanting to be criticized, teachers are reluctant to demand diligence from their students, let alone mastery of difficult material. In sum, fear of student criticism plays a major role in draining the rigor out of all post-elementary education. That fear may not cost lives in gender studies programs, but it could in medical school.

Of course, reducing time in the curriculum for science provided the opportunity to increase time for social justice. As part of a Robert Wood Johnson Foundation commentary on curricular reform in 2015, a group of behaviorist and medical educators from industry and academia shared their newfound wisdom with the world:

> [...] curricular integration aimed at advancing the impact of education will need to go well beyond basic scientists collaborating with physicians. Curricular integration means shifting learning from a focus limited to basic and/or clinical learning to this: a focus on health and well-being and what the physician *and others* together can bring to bear to improve and preserve health.

To this point, the message seems benign enough and relatively free of jargon, but the authors are just warming up:

> To this end, curricular integration must also include scientists who do not study health but who study instead the determinants of heath [sic]. Curricular integration must better connect medical faculty and trainees with other disciplines (public health, sociology, economics, engineering, and more). Curric-

ular integration must also provide the learner with a more holistic view of the patient. Integrating the social determinants, social and other sciences, and a whole-patient view is vital for students who, as residents, will likely encounter patients who are poor and underserved, whose illnesses stem from their housing, their food choices, their education— that is, social determinants of health.[27]

Having cared for many patients during my clinical career as a nephrologist, I did not need months of indoctrination in social sciences to make sure that patients could afford their medication. All I had to do was ask them if they could afford it. Those needing further assistance I sent to the social services department. Ayelet Kuper and Marcel D'Eon apparently don't agree with me. Writing in *Medical Education*, they have come to an odd way of thinking:

> Medical educators must progress beyond tinkering with the contents of the current medical curriculum and re-imagine it entirely based on the kinds of bioscientific, social scientific, and humanities-mediated knowledges that doctors need to truly enact all of their roles in the specific social, political and cultural contexts in which they work.

Kuper and D'Eon wrote this gibberish in 2010. Since then, more and more medical schools have chosen to "re-imagine" their curricula along these lines, so along the lines, in fact, that Penn introduced theirs in the 1990s. I am glad to say some faculty protested. In a recent survey on faculty response to curriculum reform, 30 percent of the schools surveyed reported faculty resistance. Here are some of their objections:

---

27. Marla Salmon et al., "Refocusing Medical Education Reform: Beyond the How," *Academic Medicine* (February 2015), https://docksci.com/refocusing-medical-education-reform-beyond-the-how_5a9a0bb-4d64ab2a4c7b97165.html.

- Faculty were opposed to reducing preclinical time.

- Basic scientists feared that they would be marginalized.

- Faculty were opposed to losing course control (basic science faculty) when clinical and basic science courses were integrated.

With the winds of change at their back, the leaders of the curriculum revision movement blew through faculty protests. While it is true that any changes in curriculum need to be approved by some vote of the faculty, typically only a small number of faculty is willing to speak up to administrators. As a result, the changes were inevitably passed and approved just about everywhere without much deference to the opposition.

The student uprisings of the late 1960s and early 1970s created a dynamic that certainly contributed to the decline in educational rigor across almost all disciplines in higher education. Now students felt empowered to demand input into the content and teaching methods in higher education. Moreover, as the rebellious students became university faculty, they tended to side with their own students in their calls for a less stressful and demanding medical school experience. Of course, curriculum changes were never promoted as less demanding but rather as more efficient and more likely to promote student "wellness."

Medical students were attracted to the idea that they would not need to spend long hours in classrooms learning the details of hard sciences like biochemistry and genetics. Somehow faculty and educational leaders convinced themselves that students could learn all they "needed" to learn in less than half the time their predecessors spent in science classes. Students, including medical students, also expected to be entertained in the classroom, not simply instructed in the necessary material.

These expectations began to drive the curriculum. Increasing time was spent in the early stages of medical school in "doing" rather than "learning." For example, in some schools, students participated in medical clinics from the first day in medical school despite having no previous training or expertise in providing any sort of medical care. This playacting was supposedly going to show them the "relevance" of their classroom work to caring for patients. Indeed, it is hard to imagine a more infantilizing activity. This approach assumes that students, who went through the effort to apply to medical school with all the required courses and exams, do not understand the role science plays in their chosen profession.

These and other such initiatives helped promote the idea that medicine was "fun." These exercises supposedly gave purpose to the classroom work that was otherwise viewed as a burden. This is not to say that so-called "active learning" is not highly useful. Students can benefit from solving problems rather than passively sitting back and listening to lectures. In an influential 2006 review in *Advances in Physiology Education*, Joel Michael documented the advantages of active learning in the sciences.

To be effective, however, sufficient time must be devoted to the problem-solving exercises. And since physiology is an amalgam of chemistry and physics, rigorous learning is required to understand the basic mechanisms of healthy organ function and disease. Participating in clinical care before learning anything about the scientific basis of clinical care is more entertainment than scholarship.

The public expects physicians in training to learn as much as they can about patient care, but the reality is quite different. The Liaison Committee on Medical Education (LCME) establishes standards for medical school accreditation and conducts intense reviews of each medical school on a periodic basis. The LCME outlines a series of "standards," or rather vague instructions, on the content of medical education. One of the standards speaks directly to still another unhelpful change in medical school curricula.

Standard 7.2 requires medical schools to educate their students about the health-related impact of socioeconomic problems with equal weight given to learning how to diagnose and treat diseases. Although the LCME gives latitude to each medical school to create curricula to achieve the goals set out in the standards, woke medical school administrators and faculty have seized the opportunity to promote an expanding curriculum in fields like social policy and gender equity. Indeed, they have created a veritable industry of race and gender-obsessed books and articles. The AMA master plan lists eighty-two references to such material, several of which are dedicated to finding and exposing otherwise unseen racism. The two titles that struck me were *Race After Technology: Abolitionist Tools for the New Jim Crow* and *Racism without Racists: Color-Blind Racism and the Persistence of Racial Inequality in America*, the latter in its fifth frightening edition.

These programs are devoted to creating cadres of young physician activists who will use the trust placed in them in their role as doctors to convince the public to adopt all sorts of Progressive schemes.

The Lancet, the prestigious British medical journal, has published lengthy articles arguing for Progressive programs to solve the world's social ills and for physicians to be key advocates for the enactment of these programs. In March 2005, the World Health Organization (WHO) established the Commission on Social Determinants of Health to support countries and global health partners in addressing the social factors leading to ill health and health inequities. After three years of study, the commission called on the medical community to do the following:

1. Improve Daily Living Conditions

2. Tackle the Inequitable Distribution of Power, Money, and Resources

3. Measure and Understand the Problem and Assess the Impact of Action[28]

---

28. "Closing the gap in a generation," *Commission on Social Determinants of Health FINAL REPORT | EXECUTIVE SUMMARY, World Health Organization,* https://www.who.int/social_determinants/final_report/csdh_finalreport_2008_execsumm.pdf.

"Tackle the inequitable distribution of power, money, and resources?" Why should students bother with a medical education when they can just read *Das Kapital*? Karl Marx would seem to have "tackled" this issue more than a century ago. For reasons never quite explained, the WHO commission proposed that teaching medical students about the social determinants of health would somehow produce their desired outcomes. Medical schools such as the University of Colorado, Harvard, Mount Sinai, and many others have already instituted curricula to teach social advocacy. Student groups like White Coats for Black Lives, when not busy attacking "cisheteropatriarchy" and other evils, played a major role in organizing the George Floyd protests.

Advocating for individual patients is, of course, an obligation for physicians. For example, persuading insurance companies to allow advanced treatments or to pay for certain expensive medications is entirely proper and within the sphere of medical care. But learning about and advocating for solutions to the "inequitable distribution of power, money, and resources," as proposed by the Commission on the Social Determinants of Health, is wildly inappropriate and an intrusion on the student's medical education. Efforts to promote these activities are mostly ineffectual, ill-informed, and doomed to failure if they have not already failed.

Chapter 11

The Ascendant Educational Class

In 2004, Kenneth Ludmerer, a noted historian of medical education, writing in the *New England Journal of Medicine*, excoriated medical schools for failing to provide the proper educational environment for students:

> Since the late 19th century, in addition to instilling high professional standards, medical education has been aimed primarily at helping medical students develop the power of critical reasoning, the capacity to generalize, the ability to acquire and evaluate information, and the intellectual tools to become lifelong learners. Accomplishing these goals requires thoughtful and personalized teaching. Instructors must generalize and synthesize, not just provide the view from their particular specialty. Students need seminars, tutorials, and individualized instruction, not lectures alone, for their reasoning powers to be developed fully. Students also need close interactions with

experienced, mature physicians in the work of patient care — and the opportunity to talk with them about that work. Such a curriculum can be constructed only if a medical faculty sufficiently values teaching to take the time to do it well. Here, medical schools have typically fallen short of their potential.

Unfortunately, they continue to fall further and further short. In the years since 2004, if anything, medical school education has been relegated to a lower priority in the world of academic medicine. Educators, meaning real teachers, have become a commodity. They are more tolerated than celebrated. The academic stars are now the high-profile clinicians and researchers who garner the publicity, clinical revenues, and research grants that are the lifeblood of academic medicine.

This is bad enough. Worse is the emergence of a progressive educational leadership class nurtured, of all places, in schools of education. An "MD" is no longer credential enough. Unknown to the public, an advanced degree from a school of education is now a requirement for those who wish to lead the educational mission at most medical schools in the United States. All politics aside, schools of education have a nationwide reputation for intellectual vacuity. "Schools of education represent the academic slums of most any college," scoffed the late Black economist Walter Williams. "American education can benefit from slum removal."

"Rigor was non-existent," said Larry Sand, who survived his school of education experience at Cal State in the 1980s. Then, in the 1990s, as Sand noted in an article for the James G. Martin Center for Academic Renewal, "[...] the fad of multiculturalism took hold [...]." Soon the fad turned "epidemic," and the 1980s began to seem like a golden age. Observed Martin, "Teachers-to-be were forced to learn about this ethnic group, that impoverished group, this sexually anomalous group, that under-represented group, etc.—all under the rubric of 'Culturally Responsive Education' (CRE)."

Schools of education have become notorious for generating flawed and unproven educational theories. Today, their graduates are busily disseminating these bad ideas throughout the medical establishment. The rot begins at the top. What follows is a sample of courses available at the Harvard Graduate School of Education:[29]

- Strategies and Policies for Educational Excellence with Equity
- Say Her Name: Gender, Race and Punishment from Tituba to Breonna Taylor
- Citizenship, Segregation, and Racial Equality in Schools
- Race and the State: The Role of Public Policy in U.S. Racial Inequality
- Educational Justice
- Preserving Privilege, Contesting Exclusion: Parents' Roles in Educational Inequality
- Race, Equity, and Leadership
- Coaching with Equity in Mind I

What is frightening is that I am not cherry-picking. I pulled the courses cited above from the first two pages of Harvard's fifteen-page online catalog. None of these courses—and precious few of the others—will equip educators to develop better doctors. Rather, newly minted EdDs will feel compelled to impose their woke ideology on medical students. Let me share a sample of

---
29. "Catalogue," Harvard Graduate School of Education.

that wokeness from Aaliyah El-Amin's course, "Educating to Transform Society: Preparing Students to Disrupt and Dismantle Racism." Here is the first thing our future educators will learn, "The persistence of injustice and oppression in the United States, specifically along racial lines is clear: Racism is a pervasive feature in American society." It would be clearer if Professor El-Amin knew the right place to put her commas.

"As a culminating project," El-Amin concludes, "students will design and if desired, implement an education and liberation based anti-racist intervention." Not surprisingly, El-Amin herself has an EdD from the Harvard Graduate School of Education. This madness is now being imposed on our medical students, and they are scarcely in a position to dissent.

Given what is learned in graduate education courses, the implementation of "modern" educational theories has failed to achieve Ludmerer's call for enhanced teaching in medical school. One source of that failure is the reliance by the education establishment on adult learning theory, a paradigm developed by American educator Malcolm Knowles more than fifty years ago. Knowles used the marvelously awkward term "andragogy" as a synonym for adult learning theory. The word is a neologism cobbled together from the Greek words for "man" and "leading." Once campus feminists realize that "andros" in Greek means "man," the word might be banned, but in the interim, andragogy boosters propose that adults, male or female, learn in ways quite distinct from the way children learn (pedagogy). This theory has been extensively applied in medical education. It consists of the following tenets, as described by Prof. John Rachal:

    — The adult learner is self-directing, needing less direction from a teacher.

    — The adult learner brings a different quality and greater volume of experience to the learning setting, which can be used as a basis for further learning.

— The adult learner approaches the learning activity on a need-to-know basis often rooted in the developmental tasks associated with his or her adult roles.

— The adult learner is problem- and task-centered.

— The adult learner may be motivated by external motivators, but the "more potent" motivators are internal such as self-esteem, recognition, greater quality of life, and greater self-confidence.

This paradigm is widely incorporated into medical education. It makes sense that an adult wishing to learn a new trade or craft would be able to set his or her learning goals. But medicine isn't plumbing. No one dies from a botched toilet repair. Medical students, for at least several years, must have their goals set for them.

Whether or not they are particularly interested in gastrointestinal physiology or neural science, students must learn the key elements of these fields. No matter what specialty of medicine they ultimately pursue, their patients may develop illnesses related to these functions. At some point in their medical training, learners might profitably set their own goals, but the first year or two or three of medical school is not that point. Students are entering a field in which they have no real sense of what is important and what their goals should be. Yet, the proponents of adult learning theory advocate for student input and evaluations as a way to plan course content.

At Penn, a committee consisting of faculty and students meets each month to review specific courses. An example of the problem of students setting goals may be seen in the reactions to a course on epidemiology and biostatistics. This topic is required learning for any physician. It is impossible to read a medical journal with any insight into the validity of a study without an appreciation for study design and data analysis.

As might be expected, students generally dislike this topic. It seems far removed from what they expected to study in medical school. They would much rather hear about diseases and therapies. Nevertheless, a course that relies on a heavy dose of statistical tests is essential. As clueless as they might be, however, students are still given the opportunity to criticize the instruction they receive and to rate the faculty. They are even given a role in determining the content of their instruction.

I have written in the medical education literature about our success in consulting with students about the effectiveness of the teaching. That is an appropriate topic for discussion. If the students did not understand a concept because it was poorly taught or if the lecturer failed to follow his own outline for a given topic, there is value in working with instructors to improve the quality of their teaching. But this is quite different from students approving the *content* of the teaching.

To be sure, many medical educators dispute this criticism. According to Dr. Stuart Goldman, who devised a new assessment model for students at Harvard Medical School, the standard pedagogic model of education is a failure:

> Most traditional evaluations are experienced by the majority of trainees as externally regulated rather than internally regulated. They do not feel "self-directed," nor do they experience the motivation for mastery as intrinsic as they would if the assessment tools were informed by adult learning theory.

Goldman rejects traditional ways of supervising and assessing student performance. As he sees things, students can monitor themselves and be better motivated to learn if they are given that power. Goldman is in good company. Here is another example of the adult learning theory of medical education from the Yale School of Medicine:

The philosophy of the Yale System of Medical Education (the Yale System), which has been in place at YSM since 1931, values medical students as mature, highly motivated, and self-directed learners. The Yale System aims to create a highly collaborative learning environment. There is a reduced emphasis on grades and no class rank to limit competition. There is a flexible curriculum to accommodate individual learning styles and allow students to pursue individual interests, with self-assessment and collaborative learning emphasized. The Yale System is considered one of the school's most powerful educational strengths.

This all sounds so good on paper that it has become the reigning philosophy in American medical education. In practice, andragogy contributes to the superficiality of the curriculum and the lax assessment of student performance. Adult learning theory may work well enough for those medical students who are self-motivated and highly intelligent. It works much less well for those who are neither. Med schools will graduate these students anyhow, thinking them "good enough." The result is a workforce that contains a sizable minority of unqualified people passing as physicians.

Adult learning theory should be viewed as a highly controversial approach to medical education. Instead, it has become the conventional wisdom for training future doctors. According to a review by Mukhalalati and Taylor in the *Journal of Medical Education and Curricular Development* in 2019, some 726 publications in the medical education literature discussed the use of adult learning theory in health-care education, almost all uncritically. Although some of these articles were directly related to Knowles's theory of andragogy, most simply spun out a related theory as if introducing a new educational mode led inevitably to improved results. This is not to say that creating a pleasant environment for learning is wrong. What is wrong is relaxing standards to conform to new theoretical formulations that are basically unproven.

Unfortunately, medical educators have largely ignored the lively academic criticism of andragogy that has emerged in other academic disciplines. In an *Adult Education Quarterly* article, John Rachal, a professor at the University of Southern Mississippi, reviewed the criticism of adult learning and attested to its weakness. Apparently, unbeknownst to medical educators, adult learning theory has caused more controversy and stirred more philosophical debate than just about any other educational model. Yet only a few studies have attempted to empirically investigate its validity. Following his review, Rachal cast doubt on the current state of adult learning orthodoxy. "Whether andragogy can serve as the unifying theory of adult education remains to be seen," he wrote defiantly.

Rachal cited Dr. D. D. Pratt, a senior scholar in medicine at the University of British Columbia. "We cannot say, with any confidence," concluded Pratt, "that andragogy has been tested and found to be, as so many have hoped, either the basis for a theory of adult learning or a unifying concept of adult education." Despite the wobbliness of theoretical andragogy, medical educators have eagerly adopted its methods. The result is a giant experiment in medical education that risks degrading the entire health-care industry.

Chapter 12

Remedial Med 101

Nothing shouts failure quite like the two words "coaching programs." In 2020, researchers at the University of Michigan conducted a survey of the thirty-three schools attending an AMA conference on the future of medical education. Nearly all had a coaching program or were developing one. Most respondents cited professional identity formation, professionalism, and academic performance as coaching goals.

At a Johns Hopkins teaching program, Ryan Graddy and colleagues, writing in the *Journal of Graduate Medical Education*, found that first-year residents in their internal medicine residency program required coaching to satisfactorily perform even basic tasks like conducting a physical examination or taking an appropriate medical history. As they touted the benefits of coaching to improve residency performance, the authors inadvertently revealed the deficiencies of even the strongest medical school graduates. The fact that med students still needed personal remediation suggests that the current educational model is not exactly firing on all cylinders.

So embedded are these programs in the curricula that almost all schools offer formal coach training. Although many respondents seemed quite pleased with their coaching programs, few of them factored in the price tag. Lo and behold, there is a big one.

If each coach supervises eight students and each school has a student cohort of four hundred and fifty students in the first three years of medical school, some fifty-six faculty would be required. If the average cost of a full-time faculty member was some $200,000 per year, and each faculty member devoted 15 percent of his or her time to coaching, the annual coaching cost for this institution would be $1.68 million, and that doesn't include the cost of administering the program or coaching the coaches.

If we need proof of the nationwide need to improve student selection and academic rigor, we need only calculate the multiple millions of dollars spent each year to correct the deficiencies of medical school curricula. Program boosters insist that coaching enhances the students' professional development. What it really does—or tries to do—is remediate obvious weaknesses throughout the curriculum. The laments of newly graduated medical students faced with the COVID-19 pandemic suggest just how consequential those weaknesses are.

In 2012, Ezekiel Emanuel and Victor Fuchs advocated for reducing medical school education to three years duration. Theirs was a response, in part, to the modeling that predicted a major shortfall of physicians in the coming years. A truncated education, it was argued, would also ease the economic burden on students.

My colleague, Dr. Gail Morrison, and I wrote a piece for the *New England Journal of Medicine* in 2013 in which we argued against this proposal. As we noted, this program had been tried in the 1950s and 1960s and was abandoned by all the schools that participated in the experiment. It was generally felt that the education was too rushed and too pressured. The students hated it, and the faculty hated it even more. Otherwise, it was a roaring success.

Past failed experiments aside, we felt that students were simply unprepared after three years to take on clinical responsibilities. We pointed to the UCSF study cited earlier. According to the study, supervisors found that even after four years of medical school, many students lacked sufficient medical knowledge to embark on a residency.

We also pointed to the experience of medical education in New Zealand. There, as here, students were not ready for substantial clinical responsibilities after three years in medical school. As in many European and English-speaking countries, medical students in New Zealand typically attend the equivalent of college for one year and then have four years of medical studies all at one institution. But the New Zealanders found that their students, after the traditional four-year curriculum, were unprepared for internships. To compensate, they added a new bridge year before students could assume independent clinical responsibility.

Importantly, too, the New Zealanders rejected the adult learning theory model of allowing students to pursue a series of elective courses to reflect their particular interests. Instead, they created an internship training year in which students are assigned to a specific hospital and, while closely supervised, act as interns with progressive clinical responsibilities. The students receive a stipend as employees. They like that.

While the enlightened New Zealanders were extending the undergraduate training time for medical students, their American counterparts sought ways to reduce training time. One of the main arguments forwarded here is that the current fourth year of medical school is a waste of time. The critics have a point.

As noted, students devote too much of their fourth year to the pursuit of a desired residency position. Some specialties are seen as more special than others. Many students, for instance, wish to train in fields such as ophthalmology, dermatology, and certain surgical specialties in which there is more demand for training positions than supply. In primary care medicine, by contrast, there is more supply than demand. The reasons for this imbalance are complex but are related to the financing of residency programs through Medicare as well as efforts to control the number of practitioners in some fields.

Despite an overall generous supply of training positions in primary care, there is a limited pathway to the more elite training programs. Ivy League medical schools and their associated hospitals and major academic centers such as Stanford, Duke, Washington University of St. Louis, and Mayo Clinic all have plentiful demand. As a result, many of the better students who choose primary care specialties such as internal medicine, pediatrics, and obstetrics and gynecology have to invest their energy in getting selected.

To improve their chances, students often spend one or two months as visiting students pursuing an elective experience in a specific program. Many of the most competitive programs encourage students to spend time with them so that program directors can evaluate the students as potential trainees. These experiences rarely provide students with in-depth clinical training. In fact, they are more like auditions. All too predictably, Penn and many medical schools engage consultants to train students on how to conduct themselves in interviews. This is something students actually could learn on YouTube and save their institution a few dollars in the process.

The rest of the fourth year may contain some required clinical courses, such as an assignment as a junior intern in which students gain progressive clinical experience for a month or two. Many schools allow students a couple of months to engage in some research activity. Although the research spruces up résumés, it is rarely anything more than pure dilettantism. Typically, too, students are given a month or two to prepare for their licensure exams. Finally, come "Match Day" in March, students receive their residency assignments and tend to disappear until graduation.

All this adds up to an educational year unworthy of the $60,000 to $70,000 billed to the students. The laxity of content and assessment in the final year reflects the attitude that medical school education is not that important. The best proof of this assertion is the indifference of the LCME, the accrediting agency for medical schools, to the content of the fourth-year curriculum.

The regularly scheduled accreditation reviews of medical schools have no stated educational requirements for the fourth year.

Those who advocate for eliminating the fourth year suggest therapy but for the wrong diagnosis. While they are correct that the fourth year could be eliminated with minimal educational impact, a wiser approach would be to improve the educational content of the fourth year. New Zealand offers a useful model with integration into the delivery of health-care services in a hospital setting. This approach could be standardized so that every student receives training in caring for critically ill patients. In the mid-twentieth century, hospitals often had "rotating" internships in which trainees spent two to three months on the core clinical activities of the major medical specialties such as obstetrics and gynecology, surgery, internal medicine, and pediatrics. Another approach could be a special track for students to pursue much more in-depth training in activities related to their chosen specialties.

The time to pursue this more rigorous path exists, but it is now being squandered. Students are spending months studying for licensure exams. They shouldn't. If, after extensive instruction, they can't pass their required exams, they should probably find a new line of work. Months spent applying for residencies should be eliminated as well. Faculty recommendations, exam scores, and Zoom interviews should do the trick. Yes, there are elements of the modern worth adapting. There just aren't many of them.

Chapter 13

First, Seize the Media

In any successful coup d'état, the insurrectionists head first for the radio and TV stations. They figure if they control the media, they control the message. The leaders of the woke coup on American medicine have taken this page right out of the revolutionary's handbook. And their message is loud and clear—the leaders of medical schools, professional societies, academic medical centers, and publications must acknowledge systemic racism in their midst and, having found it (or something that looks like it), extirpate it.

For example, in June 2020, the Association of American Medical Colleges (AAMC), an organization governed by the deans of American medical schools and the governing body for those schools, insisted, "We must acknowledge and speak out against all forms of racism, discrimination, and bias in our environments [and] in our institutions [...]." The statement went on to say, "We must move from rhetoric to action to eliminate the inequities in our care, research, and education of tomorrow's doctors."[30]

With rare exceptions, the leaders of academic medicine accepted these marching orders without resistance. They didn't have

---

30. "AAMC Statement on Police Brutality and Racism in America and Their Impact on Health," *AAMC* (June 1, 2020), https://www.aamc.org/news-insights/press-releases/aamc-statement-police-brutality-and-racism-america-and-their-impact-health.

much choice. The insurrectionists have made it clear that those who resist the revolution do not need to be heard, let alone heeded.

I received a dose of this rough medicine after I published my op-ed piece in the *Wall Street Journal*. Penn administrators debated whether my opinions had disqualified me from teaching. After much discussion, I was allowed to teach, but I was monitored for deviations from the party line. Administrators actually questioned my students as to whether I had said anything that might have upset their delicate sensibilities.

Indeed, I was being treated like a student teacher despite the fact that I had been ably teaching medical students for more than forty-five years and had the teaching awards to show for it. That my opinions on curricular content could be considered a danger to medical students reveals how far academic institutions have fallen from their traditional role as centers of inquiry and debate and how desperate they are to control the message.

Howard Bauchner, the former editor of the *Journal of the American Medical Association (JAMA)*, got to wear a dunce cap as well. In February 2021, it so happened that one of his deputy editors, Dr. Ed Livingston, conducted a podcast with Dr. Mitchell Katz, the head of the Greater New York Hospital Association, on the subject of "structural racism." Livingston acknowledged the relatively poor medical outcomes of Black patients. He suggested, however, that if "structural racism" were the cause, the system at fault was the societal one that leads to poverty, not any personal bias by physicians and administrators. Said Livingston:

> The use of race for any sort of transactional activity was made patently illegal by the civil rights legislation passed in the 1960s. Given that racism is illegal, how can it be so embedded in society that it's considered structural? As a child of the 60s, I didn't get it. I asked Dr. Katz about this concept, what it means and what needs to be done about it.

Katz knew how to play the game better than Livingston but not quite well enough. "Structural racism refers to a system in which policies or practices or how we look at people perpetuates racial inequality," said Katz. But he added, "This is not about racism—meaning someone's individual views. This is about how, as a society, we perpetuate inequality."

For his part, Livingston explained that having grown up in a Jewish household where racism was "reviled," he was always sensitive to the issue of discrimination. "Yet, I feel like I'm being told I'm a racist in the modern era, because of this whole thing about structural racism [...]."

Katz, who is also Jewish, gave a long-winded response sufficiently evasive to stay out of trouble, but Livingston came back to his larger point, an excellent one. People, he said, "are turned off by the whole structural racism phenomenon. Are there better terms we can use? Is there a better word than 'racism'?"

From the response of the woke community, you would think that Livingston had raised a Confederate flag over the offices. Trying to save his own skin, Bauchner pulled the podcast and issued this unfortunately groveling response, "Comments made in the podcast were inaccurate, offensive, hurtful, and inconsistent with the standards of JAMA. Racism and structural racism exist in the US and in health care. After careful consideration, I determined that the harms caused by the podcast outweighed any reason for the podcast to remain available on the JAMA Network."

As is inevitably the case, apologies only emboldened the activists. They forced Livingston to resign and reviled Katz for not standing up to Livingston. The AMA master plan, referenced earlier, called the posting of this podcast an "egregious, harmful error." Under pressure, *JAMA* put Bauchner on administration leave and ultimately forced his resignation. Watching the careers of these good men come undone, I began to understand why Mao's Cultural Revolution had such widespread support or at least the appearance thereof.

Feeling the heat, the AMA issued a lengthy report on its new commitment to equity. Three elements of the program are noteworthy:[31]

- Eliminating all forms of discrimination, exclusion and oppression in medical and physician education, training, hiring, matriculation and promotion supported by:

    — Mandatory anti-racism, structural competency, and equity-explicit training and competencies for all trainees and staff

    — Publicly reported equity assessments for medical schools and hospitals

- Preventing exclusion of and ensuring just representation of Black, Indigenous and Latinx people in medical school admissions as well as medical school and hospital leadership ranks.

The recommendations imply that racism exists as an endemic problem in medical care, but it falls short of indicting physicians as racist. The idea that the American health-care system is rife with racism is based on the reality of disparities in health-care outcomes for Black patients and on a collection of anecdotes in the lay press. Some research studies in the medical literature also support the accusation of racism.

The media relish stories of medical racism, true or false. Bizarrely, practitioners enable them as they did in the notorious case of Dr. Susan Moore. A Black physician, Moore claimed she was denied proper therapy for COVID-19. Dr. Moore's story was widely reported, as she made a video during her hospitalization

---

31. "American Medical Association's Plan to 'Embed Racial Justice and Advance Health Equity,'" Reddit, May 15, 2021, https://www.reddit.com/r/JordanPeterson/comments/nd6vr9/american_medical_associations_plan_to_embed/.

in which she accused her physician of ignoring her complaints of neck pain and of withholding needed analgesia. To no one's great surprise, Moore attributed her mistreatment to her White physician's racism. The video images went viral and confirmed the idea that African American patients died of COVID-19 in greater numbers, in part, because of neglect like that suffered by Dr. Moore.

Yes, Black patients have been more likely to die from COVID-19 than White patients. But the media have relentlessly covered up one of the possible reasons why—namely, obesity. Black women, for example, are nearly twice as likely to be obese as White women—58 percent to 32 percent.[32] As the CDC itself acknowledges, obesity *triples* the risk of a COVID-19 sufferer being hospitalized.[33] The CDC should be shouting this fact from the rooftops. The media should be amplifying the message. Yielding instead to the politically correct taboo against "fat-shaming," they all stay mum. Besides, to report about obesity would compromise the media's preferred theme—"racism."

The Jamaica-born Moore, who had chronic lung issues, was originally sent home but returned by ambulance to another hospital before dying on a ventilator. "Black Doctor Dies of Covid-19 After Complaining of Racist Treatment," read the *New York Times*'s predictably unhelpful headline. Moore's experience, said the *Times* without a shred of evidence, was "all too common among Black people in America." A perspective in the *New England Journal of Medicine* also suggested that Dr. Moore's death was largely due to racism.

Dr. Moore's case was a tragedy, as are all deaths related to COVID-19. But her video and her story do not validate her accusations. Her complaint was about pain and her need for pain relief. Failure to adequately treat pain and the proper treatment of pain are well-known problems in contemporary health care. It is common for patients to complain about inadequate pain relief

---

32. Marissa Seamans et al., "Exploring racial differences in the obesity gender gap," *PMC* (March 19, 2015), https://www.ncbi.nlm.nih.gov/pmc/articles/PMC4433605/.
33. "Obesity, Race/Ethnicity, and COVID-19," *CDC*, https://www.cdc.gov/obesity/data/obesity-and-covid-19.html.

in hospitals. It is hardly unique to Black patients. In one study of 1,250 hospitalized patients with pain as a major symptom, 29 percent of all patients felt their pain treatment was poor or very poor. Yet, in Dr. Moore's widely publicized case, her pain treatment became a cause célèbre for those who seek to find examples of systemic racism. The fact that her complaints had nothing to do with her death was of no importance to the media.

The chief medical officer at IU Health North Hospital, where Moore was initially treated, spoke with her. According to the *Times*, the CMO "assured her that she would get better care." As a kicker, he promised that "diversity training would be held." Patients, I suspect, would prefer their doctors spend more of their training time on "better care" than on "diversity," but for the hard core, diversity comes first.

Even the most respected newspapers abandon objectivity and allow their pages to be used for evidence-free woke propaganda. In an April 2020 *Washington Post* op-ed, Black activist Stacy Patton wrote, "Black people are at the mercy of everything that is flawed and dysfunctional about America's health-care system, which has long been shaped by racism." In May 2020, a story by reporters Sarah Gantz and Wendy Ruderman in the *Philadelphia Inquirer* was headlined, "Coronavirus has exposed deep race inequity in health care." They gave the money quote to a local pastor who insisted, "America's preexisting condition is racism, and we are seeing the fault lines of racism in real time."

In the June 10, 2021, edition of the *Philadelphia Inquirer*, the same Ms. Gantz and her editors provided a mind-numbingly typical example of big media race-baiting. The headline of a front-page article read, "How well do hospitals serve patients of color?" One might expect something about mortality rates or some other relevant parameter to be the subject of analysis. Rather, the *Inquirer* used something called the "Lown Institute Hospital Index" to rate how many Black Medicare patients are seen in each hospital compared to the number of Black patients in its "service area." Gantz might have pointed out that Dr. Lown was one of the founders of the highly partisan group, Physicians for Social Responsibility, but she didn't. Of course not.

The idea that this parameter in any way reflects racism is idiotic. Yet, after bemoaning the "deep racial inequality in the U.S. Healthcare system," Gantz and the team at the *Inquirer* affirmed the value of this index in addressing the supposed problem despite the index's admitted "shortcomings."

In the real world, if a hospital can attract more Medicare patients, it will do everything in its power to do so. Gantz pointed to a lack of insurance as a reason for hospitals to be less interested in certain patients, but the study is of well-insured Medicare patients. In this case, insurance status has nothing to do with the percentage of Black patients seen at a hospital. To equate "inclusivity," a newly important parameter in the "diversity, inclusion, equity" triad, with hospital quality or even with the care of Black patients is absurd.

In my experience in working with hospitals as the chief medical officer of a large health-care organization, the two most important determinants for choosing a hospital are rather pedestrian: how available is cheap parking and how far does one have to travel to get to the hospital. It is rare for patients to bypass a hospital nearby to get care at another facility. For example, one of the seven Penn Medicine hospitals is two blocks from the main teaching hospital. That hospital is ranked high in the Lown index, but the teaching hospital is ranked much lower. Both hospitals have Penn faculty as the physician staff. They have identical cultures and share many services and faculty. I am on the staff of both hospitals. But the hospital with the higher Lown ranking is the one closer to West Philadelphia, a predominately African American community. In this case, as in many, the Lown index is a useless measure of a hospital's "culture" but a reasonable measure of its proximity to a largely Black community. It is also a handy tool for malicious media.

In sum, the Lown index is meaningless. Yet, one hospital executive of a large suburban hospital system in Philadelphia reports that he was "sick to his stomach" that the media did not see his hospital as "inclusive." As to the data that turned his stomach, the surrounding community is 9.4 percent Black, but only 7.6 percent of the hospital's Medicare population is Black.

It is not even clear that this quantitative difference is significant. Had the executive bothered to check census data, he would have discovered that in 2019 the median age of the White population was thirty-nine. The median age of the Black population was thirty-two. Although Africans make up 13 percent of the larger population, they only account for 9 percent of those over sixty-five. Based on national figures, a community that is 9.4 percent African American should expect to have a Medicare population of 6.9 percent. In sum, it appears that the Black Medicare population at this hospital was *overrepresented*. Here's hoping that the executive settles his stomach by reading this book.

The headline of the article in question—"Racial equity is essential to hospital quality, and some in Philly are falling short, new report says"—was as irresponsible as much of the press coverage of the so-called racism of the health-care system.

Not to be outdone by the media hacks, medical journals have also yielded to the epidemic of racial self-reprisals. Many journals, including the *New England Journal of Medicine* and the *Journal of the American Medical Association*, attack the medical establishment in ways that undermine the profession. The editors, it would seem, feel the need to appear sufficiently sensitive to the feelings of their staff and readers. They have seen the ax fall on peers such as Drs. Livingston and Bauchner, cited earlier, who were not woke enough soon enough.

This fear-based editorializing is about as scientific as the *X-Files*. The editors of these prestigious medical journals seem unaware that, by welcoming unsubstantiated opinion pieces about social and political topics, they undermine their reputations.

Until recently, these journals were seen as repositories of the most rigorous and thoroughly vetted scientific efforts.

Of course, if all the allegations about racism in medicine were true and if the anecdotes of poor care or discrimination were representative of American health care, a transformation of medical education, if not a wholesale disruption of the health-care system, would be more than justified. It would be imperative. But anecdotes are not necessarily representative of anything. In fact, while there is no doubt that African American communities suffer more from COVID-19, careful studies show that the outcomes of hospitalized African American patients with COVID-19 are the same, if not superior to, that of other ethnic or racial groups.

For example, a recent study in the *Journal of the American Medical Association* about medical care in New York City, the epicenter of the initial COVID-19 outbreak in America, finds that African American patients actually had lower mortality when adjusted for factors such as age, comorbid conditions, and socio-economic factors.

This means that a poor white person with coexistent diabetes and heart disease had a greater chance of dying from COVID-19 than a Black person with the same characteristics. Other studies have also shown that while African Americans contract COVID-19 more frequently, once they do, their chances of survival are as good as, if not better than, those of White patients—once again, adjusting for the factors noted above.

Poor outcomes are more likely the result of demographic and geographic factors than of poor care. Dr. Moore's unfortunate case is typical of attacks in the press on the medical establishment for "systemic racism." Many White patients, including physician patients, gripe about their care. They have not been indoctrinated, however, to blame the quality of that care on their race. African Americans have. When the media take an anecdote of a poor outcome, attribute it to systemic racism, and don't bother with contradictory data, they inevitably heighten paranoia in the Black community.

It is hard to blame African Americans for vaccine hesitancy or other resistance to health-care recommendations when the media constantly pound them with tales of medical racism, most of them either ancient or imagined. For instance, a 2021 NPR headline reads, "In Tuskegee, Painful History Shadows Efforts To Vaccinate African Americans."[34] The study of Black syphilis patients began nearly eighty years ago, but the media will not let it go. And even NPR acknowledges the consequences of these perpetual reminders: "A lingering mistrust of the medical system makes some Black Americans more hesitant to sign up for COVID-19 vaccines." So why pound them over the head with reminders that are no longer relevant? The woke reap what they sow.

Hoping to show his commitment to anti-racism, President Joe Biden raised the specter of Tuskegee in explaining Black vaccine hesitance. Unfortunately, he got the wrong Tuskegee reference. It was, said Biden in his inimitable way, "harder to get African-Americans, initially…vaccinated, because it used to be that they experimented on them—the Tuskegee Airmen and others." Most Americans know of Tuskegee for only two things: the misguided Tuskegee experiment on Black patients and the heroic Black Tuskegee airmen of World War II fame. Biden couldn't quite sort them out. Even if he had gotten the right Tuskegee reference, what good would this reminder have accomplished?

Let me cite another everyday example, equally pernicious, of the press and woke physicians colluding to create a destructive narrative about health-care disparities. On August 10, 2021, the *Philadelphia Inquirer* ran a story headlined, "Decades of Penn research shows how structural racism affects Black children with type 1 diabetes." On seeing this, an African American parent would likely think, "Here we go again." The newspaper story tells the reader nothing about the data accumulated in decades of research but a whole lot about the opinions of two practitioners at Children's Hospital of Philadelphia (CHOP).

---

34. Debbie Elliott, "In Tuskegee, Painful History Shadows Efforts To Vaccinate African Americans," NPR, February 16, 2021, https://www.npr.org/2021/02/16/967011614/in-tuskegee-painful-history-shadows-efforts-to-vaccinate-african-americans.

Although the *Inquirer* acknowledges that "biological differences" may account for the disparity, Terri Lipman, a CHOP-based pediatric nurse practitioner, cut right to the chase. "Structural racism is really the underpinning of racial disparities," she insisted. Why this is so, the reader has no clue. Lipman also discounted the suggestion that "patients need to be better or behaviors need to change." For her, that smacks of blaming the victim. Better to ignore biology, deny patients' responsibility for their own actions, and blame White America. Upon reading this, African Americans would likely be even more distrustful of the medical establishment than they already are.

Lipman and her colleague, Colin Hawkes, clinical director of CHOP's diabetes center, also coauthored an opinion piece on structural racism in the medical journal *Pediatrics*. To reach their conclusions, they reviewed a study of patients from throughout the world as well as from the US. Nowhere in the *Inquirer* article is there any mention of the international origins of the study. Structural racism may exist in New Zealand, but their minorities are not of African descent and have had an entirely different history than American Blacks. Mentioning that the study included diverse other countries would have undermined the implication that American physicians uniquely mistreat Black children. Better to ignore that fact.

The *Inquirer* editorial, especially Lipman's killer quote, was tweeted widely and cited in other publications around the nation. What should the reporter, Sarah Gantz, have done with the story? First, she might have asked the CHOP practitioners what their data were. Given that they have "spent decades tracking childhood type 1 diabetes," she might have inquired as to whether they identified structural racism in their own backyard at CHOP? If so, what have they done to remediate it? Unfortunately, if they solved the problem of outcome disparity for Black patients, the media would not be interested. The media prefer the narrative that patients and families are victims and have little or no role in their health outcomes.

Once again, wading into the issue of disparities in health outcomes requires objectivity that escapes many physicians and clearly many reporters. I don't believe that journalists, or physicians for that matter, do a service to African Americans in the community who have children with type 1 diabetes by blindly criticizing the kind of care that is currently provided. Pointing to disparities in the outcome as prima facie evidence of so-called structural racism insults the honor of the physician and the intelligence of the patient. I know critical race theory calls for this kind of assessment, but is the theory correct? Does it help any patients? No and *no*.

The reliance on anecdotal evidence is not restricted to the lay press. Many prestigious medical journals have published editorials and perspectives that are completely anecdotal. In a perspective in the *New England Journal of Medicine* in July 2020, Dr. Michele Evans indulged in the kind of logical fallacy that passes for medical science today. "The disproportionate effects of the Covid-19 pandemic on African Americans, Latinx Americans, and Native Americans is not unforeseen," wrote Evans. "Inequities in health, health care access, and quality of care are ingrained in the U.S. health care system." As the Romans might say, *post hoc ergo propter hoc*.

These opinion pieces in the medical literature, like those in the lay press, adhere to a recurring pattern. They attribute relatively poor clinical outcomes for Black patients to physician bias and support their accusations by citing historical examples of actual racial bias, such as the Tuskegee study. Other than that study, launched eighty years ago, critics fail to identify any contemporary examples of "systemic racism" in the health-care system they criticize. Of course, if unequal poverty rates, incomes, housing, and the like are called "racism"—and no variables other than race are factored into the equation—it is a whole lot easier to find examples of "racism."

Chapter 14

Confirmation Bias

One form of bias is, in fact, epidemic in medical research today, and that is called "confirmation bias." Most, if not all, researchers devoted to examining differences in clinical care for Black and White patients are hell-bent on finding such differences and attributing those differences to racism. These research studies are used as a scientific backstop to validate anecdotal experiences.

One typical op-ed by a Black physician, this one in the *New York Times*, related how he had been witness to and recipient of "racist" slurs and taunts. In passing, he mentioned that many research studies "proved" racism exists in medicine and that racism contributed to poorer outcomes for Black patients. His own experiences are, of course, anecdotal. He cites the medical literature, however, to show how statistics support his claim that the mistreatment of Blacks is not due to chance. Of course, these studies rarely account for bias on the part of those doing the study. Researchers would have a much more "interesting" story to tell if they find evidence of discriminatory behavior than if they fail to. "Uninteresting" studies have a much harder time getting published in prestigious journals. Today, in fact, to publish an uninteresting study could cost an editor his or her job. As is painfully obvious, there is an incentive to find "racism" when investigating disparate health outcomes.

There are daunting complexities in carrying out research about the health care of African Americans, Latino populations, or other groups living in neighborhoods characterized by low incomes, high rates of violent crimes, or other such problems. Availability of health-care services, health literacy, income, social capital such as family support, marriage status, and many other demographic factors are linked to health status and outcomes of any clinical condition.

In general, groups living in zip codes with high rates of poverty have a disproportionate share of conditions such as obesity, diabetes, hypertension, and chronic heart and kidney disease. There are high rates of pregnancy complications and infant mortality as well. The fact that poverty, aside from race, is associated with worse health outcomes is well recognized.

Rigorous epidemiologic studies try to account for the impact of economic factors when assessing the outcomes. Researchers cite any number of factors as contributing to the poor health status associated with poverty. These include the stress of difficult and dangerous blue-collar jobs, the anxiety that violence evokes, the high use of tobacco and alcohol, and poor nutrition.

Today, however, researchers, even prudent ones, feel the need to hypothesize that, in addition to the burdens imposed by poverty, physicians treat Black patients differently than White patients. Study after contemporary study is flawed by the failure to interpret the bases for any observed difference in clinical outcomes properly.

Scientific inquiry requires a rigorous framework to produce studies that are reliable. One of the key tenets of science is that a competent scientist performs experiments that attempt to disprove his thesis. Einstein was one such scientist. "No amount of experimentation can ever prove me right," said he. "A single experiment can prove me wrong." If scientists fail to disprove a given theory, then that is the best support for its validity. In this way, bias in favor of a theory is reduced as much as possible. This method is not perfect, but it is the hallmark of good science. Unfortunately, most studies claiming to find racism in medical care ignore good scientific methods. The design of these studies and the interpretation of results are almost inevitably biased to find racism, and voilà—the studies usually find it.

Most studies exploring how Black patients are treated consist of a retrospective analysis. These studies usually consist of a review of medical records and an attempt to compare how frequently Black and White patients with particular diseases were referred to specialists and whether clinical outcomes varied between the racial groups.

Such studies are always limited by the uncertainty of whether there are confounding factors besides race that might explain disparate outcomes. For example, it is often impossible to determine from medical records if one cohort does poorly because its members were unwilling or unable to accept the physicians' recommendations. Patients' trust in the health-care system, their understanding of medical options, and other such factors may play an important role in any observed outcomes.

Too many researchers are indifferent to such factors. Some years back, Dr. Clive Callender, a transplant surgeon who founded the Howard University Transplant Center in 1973, launched an inquiry into the reasons why proportionately fewer Black patients receive transplanted kidneys. He and his colleagues invoked "systemic racism" as the explanation before this designation became commonplace. They specifically attributed the disparity to White doctors treating Black patients as inferiors.

Despite multiple efforts by government agencies and physician organizations throughout the nation to increase the number of Black patients receiving kidney transplants, the substantially lower number compared to White patients persists to this day.

Recent research from the Veterans Administration, whose physicians conduct more than 300 kidney transplants each year, provides some answers as to why. The VA researchers identified education, family structure, and willingness to undergo transplantation among the factors producing the disparate results. Important too was having a spouse who could support a patient through the complex treatment protocols. Lack of such family support, researchers found, tends to discourage patients from opting for surgery and the demanding medication regimen it requires.

It is no coincidence that married men of all races live longer than their unmarried peers. Black patients in the VA study had a lower rate of marriage than White patients. Without a spouse to help out—and nag as need be—many men choose an alternative treatment like dialysis therapy. Again, the evidence does not substantiate the default assumption that "racism" is the cause of a disparity in outcomes.

Studies of possible physician bias in the treatment of heart diseases often explore the referral rates of Black and White patients for invasive studies such as cardiac catheterization. If Black patients end up less frequently than White patients in the cardiac catheterization lab, this disparity, supposedly, is prima facie evidence of racism.

One of the most widely cited studies on this issue was published in 1999 in the *New England Journal of Medicine*. Investigators asked physicians attending medical conventions to agree to review simulated clinical scenarios and then make recommendations about further testing or treatment. Unlike almost all the studies using a retrospective analysis of outcomes, this study had a prospective design. The investigators used brief films of Black and White actors, men and women, complaining of chest pain. The physician volunteers were provided laboratory tests and imaging studies and asked whether they would refer each patient for further invasive testing using cardiac catheterization.

The physicians referred Black men and White men with similar complaints and lab tests for cardiac catheterization at the same frequency. However, when comparing Black women and White women with similar complaints, the White women were referred for catheterization more frequently than the Black women. The physician volunteers recommended other tests such as cardiac stress tests at equal rates for Black and White women.

This study has been cited more than four hundred times in the medical literature as clear evidence of medical racism. Whenever it is cited, the citing authors simply use it to affirm that physicians are biased against Black patients without the caveat that there was a difference only for women. But obviously, the basis for recommending catheterization went beyond race. In fact, there was literature at the time suggesting that women do less well than men in coronary bypass surgery. Valid clinical judgment rather than bias may have been at work. Current conventional wisdom, however, demands that any differences in referral patterns be attributed to systemic racism.

One of the investigators I contacted told me he had no idea why the findings only pertained to women. Again, other investigators do not hesitate to attribute the results to racism without acknowledging the crucial distinction of a gender component to the findings. Later articles could have cited this report to show that physicians treated White and Black men equally and simply reported that for some unknown reason, the results differed for women. That narrative is much less interesting than invoking systemic racism.

A carefully designed study published in the prestigious *Journal of the American College of Cardiology* in 2000 and conducted by Okelo and colleagues at Case Western Reserve School of Medicine found no differences in the pattern of referral for invasive testing when Black and White patients were rigorously matched for age, education attained, and underlying conditions. Unlike the widely cited previous study, this research has been cited only eight times in the medical literature. This sort of citation bias helps explain the myth that Black patients are subject to poor medical care.

Another widely cited study published in the *New England Journal of Medicine* found that Black patients treated by a cohort of cardiologists were referred less frequently than White patients for invasive heart procedures. But the study was designed to test whether Black cardiologists would refer Black patients more frequently to get the extensive tests compared to White cardiologists. The study found no difference between the two cardiologist groups. Both White and Black cardiologists tended to act similarly and referred Black patients with chest pain less frequently than White patients.

One supposes the disparity may be explained by racist tendencies in both cohorts of cardiologists, but clearly, there is more going on here than bias against Black patients. Moreover, other investigators that cite these results rarely if ever bother to describe the nuances of the studies or the important point that the skin color of the cardiologist did not explain the outcomes. This study could be cited as proving that White and Black cardiologists treat patients similarly, but that is a much less compelling narrative than that Black patients are less frequently referred for cardiac catheterization.

It is also instructive that in this study, as well as in most others that assess conscious or unconscious bias, investigators fail to question the treating physicians. It might help to know why they treated their patients the way they did. Investigators also fail to get detailed demographic data about health literacy and social support that might explain patient reluctance to undergo invasive testing. Finally, most studies assume that more testing and more cardiac procedures represent better care for heart patients.

That is not necessarily so. Consider an alternate hypothesis: Physicians perceive that patients with more social capital, better family support systems, and higher levels of trust in the medical establishment will expect more treatments and therapeutic interventions. While these interventions may be more rewarding for physicians, they may not be in the patients' best interests. Do physicians tend to treat Black patients more rationally than White patients? Possibly, yes.

There is quite a bit of evidence supporting the concept that "overtreatment" may explain any perceived disparities. In a recent study reported in the *Journal of the American Medical Association*, researchers surveyed some 2,100 physicians on the question of how much medical care is unnecessary. On average, they estimated that more than 20 percent of overall medical care was unnecessary, including 22 percent of prescription medications, roughly 25 percent of tests, and 11 percent of procedures. Some 85 percent of the physicians cited fear of a malpractice suit as one reason for the overtreatment. The second most commonly cited reason, and the one most relevant to this discussion, was "patient pressure/request" at 59 percent.

Yet in the medical literature on racial disparities, researchers start with the assumption that Black patients are undertreated, not that White patients are overtreated, in part perhaps because of the demands of White patients. Interesting support for this idea comes from a study in the cardiology literature. The study found the mortality rate in major academic medical centers for cardiac patients fell dramatically during the weeks that the major cardiology societies held their national meetings. At these times, the senior cardiologists were at the conferences rather than at the bedsides of their patients.

Their younger colleagues, as it turned out, were left to care for patients at the home institutions and were less likely to perform potentially dangerous cardiac procedures. The holiday from overtreatment benefited the patients. It bears repeating that the confirmation bias of investigators plays a major, perhaps dominant, role in interpreting studies that find disparate results between Black and White patients.

In reviewing the literature, I am astounded at just how much labor and money have been wasted in this perverse effort to find racism in the medical system. In all the literature I reviewed, I found not a single instance in which the researchers' "discovery" benefited a single patient. These studies may have helped the researchers advance their careers—publishing is essential in academic medicine—but they have also helped aggravate the racial divide.

Chapter 15

Saving the World

There is no optic quite as compelling as that of white-coated young men and women marching to end some injustice or another. The public sees the marchers as trustworthy, but in truth, their opinions have no more validity than that of any other nonexpert. They are simply trading on the physician's professional mystique.

No longer willing to save their patients or able to save their communities, Progressive physicians have decided to save the world, starting with their students in medical school. Given how the academic world has adopted many of the Left's pet issues, courses on the remarkably shaky science of climate change were inevitable. To be sure, we have been teaching about the effect of climate on health for years, including coursework on major tropical diseases and disorders related to high ambient temperatures, not to mention a little practical training on heatstrokes, frostbite, and the like.

Now, however, courses on climate have shifted from the therapeutic to the political. Educators hope future physicians will advocate for altered lifestyles to accommodate the fossil-fuel-free agenda. An article in the *Wall Street Journal* in 2019 reported that nearly two hundred medical schools had agreed to introduce courses about climate change into their curricula.

Recall, however, that as late as 1975, the *New York Times* was reporting, "Major Cooling May Be Ahead." By 1988, NASA decided that warming was the problem, not cooling. But a lengthy "hiatus" in temperature rise caused the ideologues to shift the term of art from "global warming" to "climate change." In much the same way, the Left shifted the terminology from "affirmative action" to "diversity," and no one was supposed to notice. In truth, early twentieth-century medical science was more scientifically sound than is early twenty-first-century climate science.

The shakiness of the science notwithstanding, medical educators at Georgetown University School of Medicine titled a 2018 *Academic Medicine* article, "It's Time for Medical Schools to Introduce Climate Change Into Their Curricula." Their proposal called for "participation in global health and sustainability initiatives." They hoped this initiative would achieve, among other supposed benefits, "locally sourced, plant-based diets."

The authors are quite open about their belief that physicians make attractive messengers for their Progressive-flavored approach to this contentious issue. In fact, they specifically endorse an advocacy agenda in the curriculum, urging "liais[on] with affiliated hospital[s] to explore green energy and related initiatives, identif[ication] and liais[on] with social justice clubs […]." Hoping to propagandize the young and the clueless, they urge their readers to "create and mobilize student groups, and use advocacy talking point resources, such as EcoAmerica's Climate for Health talking points." One of those talking points relates to mental health. "Direct and gradual physical impacts of climate change on the environment, society, and infrastructure," the authors insisted, "can lead to trauma, shock, stress, anxiety, depression, and other mental health impacts."

The source of this rather fantastic notion that climate change is a mental health problem is a 2016 US government publication that makes the following claim:

> The threat of climate change is a key psychological and emotional stressor. Individuals and communities are affected both by direct experience of local events attributed to climate change and by exposure to information regarding climate change and its effects.[35]

As should be obvious, it is not the ambient temperature that is the problem. It is the scaremongering about climate change—the "exposure to information"—that is the source of emotional distress. No, what is causing anxiety today is a steady diet of apocalypse being force-fed by cranks like Greta Thunberg. "Yet you all come to us young people for hope," said the ever-doleful teenager. "How dare you! You have stolen my dreams and my childhood with your empty words. And yet I'm one of the lucky ones. People are suffering." Until Ms. Thunberg passes a course in the thermodynamics of the earth's atmosphere, I don't think we should rely too heavily on her assessments.

Initiatives like the Georgetown proposal to include climate change in the medical school curriculum reveal the true intent of social justice training. The goal is to produce advocates for progressive-favored solutions to social problems, all the better, the AMA master plan tells us, to "address the broader issues of the climate, societal norms, macroeconomic social/health policies, and the systems of power that shape social hierarchy and gradients." By identifying capitalism as the source of the world's alleged poor health, activists seek to co-opt the medical field in the service of a Marxist agenda. In fact, the environmental movement is little more than a front for this anti-capitalist crusade.

As previously noted, the idea that physicians have a role to play in nonmedical social issues harkens back to social movements arising after World War II. Some physicians seem to be unable to control the impulse to trade on the trust of the public and advo-

---
35. Reynard Loki, "9 ways climate change is making us sick," *Salon*, April 16, 2016, https://www.salon.com/2016/04/16/9_ways_climate_change_is_making_us_sick_partner/.

cate for certain nonmedical issues. They are inclined as well to turn issues that are political or even ideological into medical issues.

Physicians for Social Responsibility (PSR) helped pioneer the field of medical meddling. In 1961, a group of academic physicians launched PSR in Boston and promptly began a quixotic effort to ban nuclear weapons. The group originally based its advocacy on the finding of strontium 90, a radioactive isotope derived from atmospheric nuclear testing, in children's teeth. The organization wrote position papers, held symposia, and eventually bagged a share of two Nobel Peace Prizes. The rationale for the 2017 award was PSR's efforts to avoid nuclear proliferation and nuclear testing. The fact that a group of physicians at Harvard Medical School thought it a good idea for the US and Russia to scrap their nuclear weapons appears to have swayed not a single person in power. The group's lack of success did not apparently faze the Nobel committee.

No one argues for the proliferation of nuclear weapons. If somehow the organization helped limit the nuclear spread, its work might have been useful. But it wasn't. The group quickly sputtered and died. But in 1973, Dr. Arnold Relman, then editor of the *New England Journal of Medicine*, encouraged Dr. Helen Caldicott to begin a global campaign against all things nuclear. She and others used the failed PSR as a shell organization to launch their new advocacy against peaceful nuclear energy. After all, both nuclear weapons and nuclear energy have the word "nuclear" in their title.

After many years of opposing nuclear power plants, the organization expanded its partisan focus and began to advocate against any fossil fuels, their current main target. They have again wrapped themselves in their white coats to specifically argue against fracking or unconventional drilling methods for natural gas. As physicians, of course, they claim to see health risks where others might not.

Unable to ever prove that nuclear power plants were linked to medical illnesses, the physicians turned their attention to fracking, arguing that regions that contain fracking gas wells suffer higher rates of cancer, hypertension, respiratory illnesses, and other chronic diseases. The fact that physicians are advocating against this activity and using medical issues as the basis of their advocacy is powerful and likely to sway public opinion and legislative agendas. Their arguments are also unsubstantiated and threaten the legitimacy of physician advocacy about real medical issues. Here is a press release from PSR in March 2021:

> As incontrovertible evidence of harm from fracking mounts and more health professionals raise the alarm, the fracking debate is taking place within an altered landscape. Today, as a growing body of scientific evidence confirms demonstrable health risks and harms from drilling and fracking operations and their attendant infrastructure, calls from the medical community for health-protective policies are growing louder.

It turns out the evidence is hardly incontrovertible: In 2019, Bamber and colleagues from the Colorado Department of Health and Environment and the Pennsylvania Department of Health found twenty studies on the purported health effects of fracking and wrote a definitive review of the scientific literature on the topic. These experts in epidemiology, free of any conflicts of interest, applied rigorous criteria to examine the validity of the studies. They did find limited evidence of asthma exacerbation. But for thirty-two other negative health outcomes claimed by PSR and others, they found "conflicting evidence (mixed), insufficient evidence, or in some cases, a lack of evidence of the possibility for harmful health effects."

PSR took on fracking less because of health concerns, less even because of environmental concerns, than because of political considerations. Pulling their marching orders from the Progressive playbook, PSR leaders zeroed in on climate change as an advocacy target. No surprise here. To help kill the fossil fuel industry, PSR has been playing the doctor card. But the hysteria that PSR induces in communities that are proximate to gas fields is simply unsupported by hard scientific data. Rather, it is driven by groupthink that all fossil fuels are evil and must be eliminated. Fracking may turn out to be a real health threat, but there is no solid evidence that it is. The debate is no place for a partisan physician organization with zero expertise in gas drilling, atmospheric thermodynamics, or, as it turns out, rigorous epidemiologic investigations.

PSR has not approached the question of fracking from a dispassionate, scientific perspective. Rather, it adopted a purely ideological view of a complex and vitally important issue for the economic well-being of communities. Physician groups with a superficial grasp of a nonmedical issue undermine the credibility of the profession when they attempt to impose their ideology on others, especially those who might suffer as a result of their ignorance.

Speaking of superficial understanding, PSR is still trying to eliminate nuclear weapons. In August 2021, two "intrepid PSR Nuclear Weapons Abolition Program interns" coordinated PSR's commemoration of the bombings of Hiroshima and Nagasaki. The PSR commemoration, its website tells us, was an attempt "to bring us all back to the center of this mission—to abolish nuclear weapons so that what happened in August, 1945 in Japan will never happen again."

Well, it hasn't happened again. Nor has there been a world war since 1945, one could argue, because of what happened in Hiroshima and Nagasaki. PSR had zero effect on this outcome. "We must prevent what we cannot cure" is the group's motto, but a more useful motto might be, "God, grant me the serenity to accept the things I cannot change, the courage to change the things I can, and the wisdom to know the difference."

Chapter 16

Weaponizing Medicine

If Hippocrates thought that the mission of the doctor was to "help the sick," today's interpreters of his oath have added a pledge, namely to "remain a member of society, with special obligations to all my fellow human beings, those sound of mind and body as well as the infirm." This seemingly innocuous addendum, developed by the medical ethicist Dr. Louis Lasagna in 1948, represented a sea change in the role of physicians.

Particularly important is the phrase, "those sound of mind and body." That command extends the physician's responsibility to the entire community as if community outreach were a natural extension of the role of the healer of the sick. Such a role assumes expertise on the physician's part to negotiate the complexities of community life. That presumed expertise, in turn, justifies physician involvement in the lives of healthy citizens.

Doctors are sometimes accused of being arrogant. Dr. Lasagna justified the accusation. What aspect of modern life is outside the bounds of the "special obligation" asserted in the revised oath? As will be seen, just about none. Many young physicians and medical students see poverty, housing, police policies, incarceration rates, climate, and gun control as legitimate concerns of the medical profession. This expanded role for physicians is the rationale for the proposed transformation in medical education. Medical students are not being educated in the complexities of social policy. They are being indoctrinated. Once programmed, they can leverage the trust placed in physicians to advocate for a variety of progressive policies that have never worked anywhere. That is certainly the expectation.

In the way of example, in April 2014, the American College of Physicians (ACP), the second-largest professional medical society in the United States, issued a report on gun control and gun violence in its own journal, the *Annals of Internal Medicine*. The policy piece had the patina of careful research, but the authors were physicians who had no expertise. The article read like a wish list of liberal talking points. The subjects ranged from the marginally relevant—how physicians should talk to patients about guns in the home—to the wildly irrelevant, including specific recommendations about concealed carry permits and so-called "assault weapons." Any Democratic politician could have written the article as it encompassed just about every conceivable political strategy to control gun sales and ownership.

The National Rifle Association (NRA) attacked the ACP policy paper as naive and often incorrect. A gun owner, for instance, who reads that the ACP wants to ban "firearms that have features designed to increase their rapid killing capacity (often called 'assault weapons' or semi-automatic weapons)" has to scratch his head. Just about every pistol manufactured in the last century is semiautomatic. The authors probably meant "automatic."

"This position paper," countered the NRA, "leaves one wondering if the authors reviewed the evidence, or just found works that suited their needs. For all of the bluster about their own important role in the anti-gun movement and all of the misuse of research findings, the ACP makes one thing clear: they respect their own rights and opinions far more than they do those of law-abiding gun owners." Not without reason, The NRA urged the ACP to "stay in your lane."

That recommendation was like catnip for anti-gun activists, prompting a renewed physician movement called #ThisIsOurLane." It is unlikely the ACP policy paper changed a single mind, but it did succeed in alienating millions of gun owners. Worse, this investment in physician time cured not a single patient of anything, not even of a gunshot wound.

Many physician groups, including the American Academy of Family Physicians and the American Academy of Pediatrics, came to the ACP's defense. They asserted that since physicians must deal with the trauma of gun violence, they have the right to express their views on gun regulation. But exactly what is the "lane" that the ACP and other medical groups should be in? One could argue that physician groups might legitimately issue reminders that there is a greater risk of self-harm if patients with psychiatric disorders own guns or live in homes where guns are available. But the ACP cannot authoritatively express opinions about the ideal number of cartridges in a magazine or the efficacy of armor-piercing bullets.

For example, the ACP, in its review of the literature on gun violence in 2014, suggested that concealed carry is associated with increased crime. But Romero and colleagues, in a 2003 study in the journal *Injury Prevention*, used law enforcement databases to show that there was no increase in crime in counties allowing concealed carry. While the ACP acknowledged this study, the authors of the policy paper nonetheless recommended that physicians advocate for laws that prohibit concealed carry permits. Why?

While this is but one of the many recommendations made by the ACP regarding gun ownership and gun legislation, ignoring data to promote a political agenda is unacceptable for a medical organization. Surveys by Harvard and Northeastern University suggest that 40 percent of American householders own a gun. While some percent of the public may support the ACP position, millions of gun owners must resent being hectored by physician groups about their constitutionally sanctioned rights. Given that trust is an important component of the patient-physician relationship, ACP's unnecessary interference is a sure way to erode that trust.

While the public generally views physicians as trustworthy, the assessment is not universal. In a Pew Research Center poll from 2019, a majority of Americans—57 percent—said that medical doctors care about the best interests of their patients all or most of the time. On the downside, 42 percent said physicians care some, a little, or none of the time. Only half believe physicians provide fair and accurate information all or most of the time.

Trust is expended by making recommendations that are not based on observed facts. Moreover, if the goal of the ACP is to prod physicians to discuss gun violence with their patients, the effort is not likely to be fruitful. Young men on the margins of society are the most likely to be involved in violence, with guns or without. They are also the least likely to visit a physician, at least until they are wheeled into the ER. The frequent questioning about gun ownership advocated by the ACP is infinitely more likely to annoy patients than dissuade them from shooting their neighbor.

Taking on political issues without expertise or experience makes physicians look amateurish and unscientific. No doubt, organized physician backing of a particular political position might strengthen support for that position. But if the advocacy is tarnished by ineffectiveness and error, it will lead to frustration, wasted time, and a loss of professional prestige.

Since the ACP published its position paper on gun control, the number of homicides in the United States rose from 14,164 in 2014 to 16,425 in 2019. That increase had everything to do with the effect on policing of Michael Brown's death in Ferguson months after the ACP paper was published—criminologists call the surge the "Ferguson effect"—and nothing to do with increased gun ownership. In 2020, more than 19,000 Americans were murdered, an unprecedented 30 percent year-to-year spike prompted in no small part by the Left's reaction to the death of George Floyd. If the ACP really wants to control violence, a meeting with Antifa and Black Lives Matter might accomplish more than a position paper.

This new orientation is, for the most part, a delusion. Physicians have no agency nor serious training in any sphere of civic life beyond medicine. The urge to meddle arises in large part from a false assumption that medicine and public health are tightly linked fields and that physicians, by dint of their medical training, have expertise in public policy or social work.

A statement issued by the American Public Health Association offers a clear delineation of the proper role of the physician in regard to public health: "While a doctor treats people who are sick, those of us working in public health try to prevent people from getting sick or injured in the first place. We also promote wellness by encouraging healthy behaviors."

Degrees in the field of public health are distinct from degrees granted to physicians. Many public health specialists do not have MD degrees. As a corollary, physicians receive virtually no training in public health. The current and past presidents of the American Public Health Association are not physicians. The technologies and goals of each field are quite distinct. Public health officials are often trained in social work and nutrition.

As we've seen, however, a lack of expertise does not stop physicians and physician groups from adopting advocacy policies. Nor does it stop medical schools from introducing curricula on advocacy. Each is an amateurish attempt to extend the scope of practice and appropriate the domain of public health.

Perhaps the most consequential example of physicians straying from their lane occurred during the COVID-19 pandemic. The experts that the government and the media sought for advice were infectious disease physicians such as Anthony Fauci of the National Institutes of Health (NIH), the CDC's Robert Redfield, and Dr. Peter Hotez of the Baylor College of Medicine. They and dozens of other infectious disease specialists became daily television fixtures. And their advice was pivotal in the decisions to lock down society in the early days of the pandemic. The problem was that they have little, if any, formal training in epidemiology, forecasting models, public policy, or social sciences. Despite these limitations, they showed an unsettling eagerness to make decisions affecting the freedom and economic futures of the American people.

Dr. Michael Osterholm is an MD but with a master's degree in public health. He is a member of the Biden administration's COVID-19 task force and has been a strong public voice through multiple media appearances. His views have sharply contrasted with those of the Fauci, Birx, Redfield group of infectious disease experts. Osterholm has seriously questioned the validity of models and their unfortunate use in guiding public policy.

Models are only as useful as the data sets used to construct them. Osterholm pointed out early in the epidemic that only by combining multiple models could researchers hope to provide reliable information. Osterholm also felt that, once vaccinated, individuals should be allowed the freedom to visit relatives and to travel, a more realistic recommendation than the continued focus on restrictions raised by infectious disease experts like Fauci.

Here, too, we see that medical training and research experience do not make physicians experts even in related fields such as epidemiology or public health policy. The early misdirection on the value of wearing masks, for instance, created ongoing uncertainty. So did the insistence on social distancing and lockdowns. Other than damaging the nation's economy and mental health, these mandates seemed to have had no better effect when enforced than when not. Less restrictive states and countries often fared as well or better than the highly restrictive ones. For instance, Oregon, a "blue" state with mask mandates and high vaccination rates, and Hawaii, an even bluer state, have had a surge in cases of the COVID-19 delta strain comparable to that of Texas and Florida with their freedom-loving governors.

An advanced degree in public health might not guarantee a more successful approach to the epidemic, but the lack of training on the social and economic aspects of pandemics is a clear deficiency in the education of those attempting to guide the nation. That training requires at least a year of coursework. More advanced training requires a two- to three-year commitment. Clearly, a knowledge of infectious diseases, treatment protocols, and vaccinology is a necessary qualification to advise the government during a pandemic, but it is not sufficient.

President Trump's advisers made crucial mistakes, particularly in their reliance on a flawed model to project the impact of COVID-19, a mistake that public health officials such as Gregg Gonsalves, a professor of public health at Yale, recognized early in 2020. Once more, physicians straying out of their lane further undermined patients' trust. Moreover, the failure of certain officials to communicate honestly with the public played into the surprising partisan divide over just about every component of the public response to COVID-19.

The pandemic offered one seriously unfortunate example of the risks physicians run when they attempt to project their medical credibility into areas that are outside their training or expertise. Moreover, if they manifest clear affinity to one political ideology—as Fauci did even when working under Trump—they risk undermining American morale and cohesion. Our nation needs to have physicians they can trust. This can only occur if physicians are worthy of that trust. Telling the public that masks were unnecessary because of a fear of insufficient supply for health-care workers followed by pleas for universal mask-wearing was a public relations disaster from which we have yet to recover. We expect politicians to lie. We expect physicians to tell the truth.

Chapter 17

Faking the Grade

In training less competent physicians than in previous eras, educators need to ask themselves two questions. First, in the effort to keep marginal students in school, how good are the tools used to assess them? Second, what is the impact of passing a larger pool of marginal students through medical school, into post-graduate training programs, and eventually into clinical practice?

Today, the criteria used for assessing whether students should advance from year to year in medical school are dismayingly lax. As previously described, the time spent in the preclinical period has been drastically curtailed in the past two decades. But the basic structure remains the same: lectures, some small group sessions to discuss the lecture content and provide clinical context to the material, and a written examination. At Penn, and at most medical schools, there are virtually no reading assignments. Exams are based almost exclusively on the lecture material. Rather than having to assimilate and integrate new material, students only need to study their notes to pass exams. Students are not even required to attend most lectures. All are livestreamed or taped.

Exams typically consist of one or two questions on topics extracted from each lecture. Each course leader then conducts a "review" of "key" topics further defining the material covered on the exam. If an exam produces unusually low average scores, teachers blame not the students but the test and lower the score needed to pass. There is no real competition among students as there is no limit on the percentage of students that can pass. Given that students generally know which topics they are to be tested on, they have to try hard to fail. The average grade on most of the exams is in the 90 percent range. The "exceptional" student is the one that manages to score below the 70 percent needed to pass.

The exams themselves are flawed. Multiple-choice tests encourage short-term memorization of facts rather than a mastery of the key concepts needed to understand future advances in medicine. This style of teaching and testing—no reading assignments, no testing on outside material—fails to encourage good students or weed out the bad ones.

Today, to fail a test is no big deal. Students are typically reexamined on the very same questions they failed to answer correctly. In one-on-one coaching sessions, the course director reviews the incorrect answers in preparation for a retest. If students fail the retest, they are given further opportunities to remediate, often by writing an essay or taking an oral exam on the topics they failed in the previous remediation efforts. We're used to remedial reading and writing programs, but few laypeople know about remedial doctoring. The medical establishment would just as soon keep it that way.

Today, students and faculty both would strongly resist a more robust response to poor performance. Everyone understands the rules of the game: Students are supposed to pass. More than one exam failure brings scrutiny on the student and perhaps probation. The clearly delineated exam content makes multiple failures nearly impossible, but even should a student fail, the student is given the opportunity to repeat the entire year. To fail medical school, a student has to really want to fail.

Even if the student doesn't care much about passing, failing is not easy. To get dismissed, the student has to fail repeated courses, then fail repeated remediations, and perhaps even fail a repeated year. This actually happened to a few students during the twelve years of my time as associate dean.

Numerical grades are recorded in some schools, but as reported in a 2015 survey, student transcripts record only a "pass/fail" grade in more than 70 percent of all medical schools. Despite the lax standards for passing the preclinical portion, students and many faculty have strongly resisted numerical grades. Student leaders have told me that eliminating grades reduced the stress that comes with competition. The fact that competition can inspire students to study more intensely for exams did not enter into their thinking.

Most faculty supported pass/fail as well. They insist that nurturing students is more important than challenging them. (Plus, multiple-choice tests are easier to grade.) Passing grades also lead to faculty popularity. In sum, many educators, perhaps most, are willing to sacrifice meritocracy for equity. No one will notice—champions of meritocracy, after all, make little noise. They rarely occupy faculty offices or demand anyone's termination. There is, however, a downside to this laxity, at least for future patients. Avoiding the stress and competition engendered by class ranking makes it hard for educators to identify the most talented students for the most competitive training positions.

During the clinical portion of a student's training, it is more difficult for educators to manage outcomes. Assessment is subject to bias by graders and to uncontrollable variables, such as the clinical unit in which a student is assigned. To allow adequate direct experience with patient care, only one or two students can be assigned to any clinical site. This leads to great variability in the educational experience.

Students are assessed in clinical settings by the interns and residents with whom they work closely. Inevitably, the personalities and attitudes of both the graders and the students affect the analysis of a given student's performance. While structured assessments help in reducing bias, they cannot eliminate it. Moreover, variability in the patients the students encounter can produce great variability in the students' performance. An articulate patient, for instance, can dramatically enhance a student's ability to transmit the patient's condition to faculty supervisors.

In recent years, a standardized exam has been used to assess each clinical experience. The National Board of Medical Examiners (NBME), the same agency that produces licensure examinations, designs the exam. Unfortunately, this exam is also graded as "pass/fail" in most medical schools. Worse, the passing grade is set to include the upper 90th percentile of all medical students taking the exam. This minimal performance level is the one recommended by NBME. To fail a so-called "shelf" or subject exam takes work. Most of those who failed simply refused to study. The one favorable aspect of the shelf exam is that it does force students to study topics that may not be addressed in their teaching sessions or on their clinical rotations.

The entire preclinical and clinical assessment system shows that the standard for passing courses in medical school is shockingly low. Educators will claim that since the admission standards are so high, all students are capable of succeeding and that only nonacademic issues could prevent completion of the course of study. But compromises in admission criteria and laxity in testing standards allow more weak students to complete medical school than just a generation ago.

Not everyone agrees with me. To be sure, all students must pass the United States Medical Licensing Examination (USMLE). Produced by the NBME, this licensure exam serves in all fifty states as the basis for granting state licenses to practice medicine. Some states also require additional qualifications, such as an acceptable interview.

The exam has three parts. The first is administered after two years of medical school and is based on basic science topics. Part two is taken after the third year of medical school and has a greater clinical focus. Part two previously contained a clinical skills and communication skills component using actors who portrayed patients. The COVID-19 pandemic interrupted this component, and it is now eliminated from the battery of testing. Part three is administered during the internship year and tests broad areas of medical practice.

To pass, a student must correctly answer 70 percent of the questions. The passage rate on this exam has increased over the last thirty years. In 1993, 91 percent of students passed part one, and 93 percent of students taking part two for the first time passed the exam. In 2019, 98 percent of students passed these exams.

Although we would like to think that improvement in the passing rate was due to improved medical school education, this is likely a false hope. Increased familiarity with the test materials and intense test preparation almost assuredly account for the better numbers.

Then, too, a test preparation industry now services medical students for every standardized test they encounter. Kaplan, Summer, UWorld, First Aid, Gold USMLE, Master the Boards, and many other services prepare students for the exams. "We are the top-rated RAPID REVIEW of USMLE Step 1, Step 2 CK, and Step 3 course providers with a 99% pass rate for the 2020 USMLE exams," boasts the copywriter for Gold USMLE. "We have had success with several medical students from across the world that are currently in residency and practicing in their field." Somehow, I don't find this reassuring.

One of the programs, UWorld, supplies students with thousands of test questions both for the subject exams and the licensure exams. It is rumored that students memorize questions from supposedly secure exams and supply them to the various preparation companies. Reportedly, most medical students in the United States subscribe to the UWorld program. Studying no longer means reading textbooks and developing an orderly approach to thinking about disease syndromes and their mechanisms. The current approach is to digest factoids by answering hundreds of test questions. Only when one answers a question incorrectly is there any need to review the subject matter.

Given that virtually all American medical students pass the licensure exams, it is impossible to identify risk factors for future failure with any reliability. It is useful to contrast the experience of medical students having a 2 percent chance of failing to qualify for licensure with a nursing student's 12 percent chance. Nurses often do not engage in the intense preparation for the exams that medical students do. If they did, it is likely that they would have a lower failure rate as well.

As a case in point, Kaplan advertises a sixfold greater chance of passing the nursing licensure exam for students that complete their preparatory course. That may be accurate or close to it. In a careful analysis conducted at Georgia College & State University School of Nursing, the class pass rate increased from 73 percent to 88 percent by initiating specific preparatory training for the exam.

The Georgia results support the thesis that the improvement in medical student pass rates most likely reflects exam preparation rather than mastery of essential knowledge. As educators have lowered the standards for acceptance into medical school and have reduced the rigor of student assessments, students now compensate by devoting maximal effort to exam preparation. Despite the gaudy pass numbers, it is more likely now than ever that marginal students can graduate medical school and enter the physician workforce.

The relaxation of standards affects all students, not just minorities admitted in the name of diversity. Low standards undermine the virtues—persistence, resilience, diligence, and a strong work ethic—historically associated with medical education. The fault lies not so much with the students as with the educators and accrediting agencies. The educators need to be liked more than they need to be respected. Feeding off this need, the accreditors require schools to develop extensive remediation programs for students who are academically underperforming. The relationship among these entities is not unlike that among subprime borrowers, the bankers that met their minority quotas by making unwise loans, and the accrediting agencies that approved the bundling of these loans. We know what happened in 2008. It should serve as a lesson.

Leaders in the various postgraduate residency training programs recognize the problem of lowered standards, especially the difficulty in identifying those students who will not perform well in residency. Some fields of medicine like neurosurgery, ophthalmology, and radiology have reserved training positions for the brightest and most academically successful students. Physicians in these fields are particularly alert to the dangers involved in downgrading merit for the benefit of equity. Some have publicly expressed their resistance to sacrificing quality for diversity. After all, a great deal of data confirms that superior performance in medical school and higher scores on standardized tests will predict strong performance among advanced trainees.

As recognized for many years, however, a pass/fail grading system will limit these specialists' ability to identify superior students. For example, more than forty years ago, the University of Virginia did a study that was reported in the *New England Journal of Medicine*. Researchers compared the performance of surgical residents who graduated from schools that graded their graduates to those coming from schools that followed the pass/fail approach. There were not many of the latter at the time. Judged on their medical competence and professionalism, the graded students performed significantly better than the pass/fail students. No resident from a pass/fail institution ranked above the 87th percentile. The pass/fail students did, however, account for 82 percent of those ranking below the 15th percentile. The authors were clear in their findings:

> A residency training program that seeks excellence among its trainees would do well to select preferentially students who apply from medical schools providing a specific class standing as part of the total evaluation of the student. It is suggested that the pass/fail controversy is symbolic of the erosion of standards that inevitably occurs when the university becomes involved in transient sociopolitical turmoil.

Forty-plus years later, that "transient sociopolitical turmoil" has become permanent sociopolitical turmoil. Studies conducted in training programs in otolaryngology, orthopedic surgery, radiology, internal medicine, and other disciplines consistently show that performance on the USMLE Step 1 exam predicts performance in residency programs. The higher the numerical score, the better, on average, the subsequent performance.

Over time, that score became the most important tool for assessing candidates for selection into the most competitive programs and disciplines. In a 2018 survey, training program directors in surgery confirmed that the score on the USMLE Step 1 exam was their key screening tool. They used it to determine which applicants should be invited for interviews, a key step in acceptance into these programs.

Despite the obvious value of recording numerical scores, a drastic change was in the works. In August 2019, representatives of five leading medical groups—the AAMC, the AMA, the Educational Commission for Foreign Medical Graduates, and the two groups that oversee the USMLE, the Federation of State Medical Boards (FSMB) and the National Board of Medical Examiners (NBME)—met to review the recommendations of still another conference, that being the Invitational Conference on the USMLE exam. As if to prove the folly of rule by committee, this august group adopted a new policy to eliminate ranked scoring and report the results of the Step 1 exam as pass/fail.

The rationale for this new, anti-meritocratic policy nicely summarizes the wholesale surrender to millennial fragility and the mindlessly woke worldview of today's educational leaders. The decision-makers asserted that the old system of reporting scores provoked great anxiety among the students and that it seemed unfair that one exam should have so much influence. Those concerns aired, the conveners got down to the real reason grading had to go: "Among self-identified racial groups, research shows that white students perform higher on the USMLE than any other group." Their goal, of course, was "to minimize those racial differences."

It was that simple. The solution to the fact that White students score better on the exam was to eliminate reporting scores. This makes about as much sense as Major League Baseball eliminating batting averages to assure that no ethnic cohort outperforms the others. To their credit, some training programs directors rejected this new policy. In 2019, writing in the journal *Academic Radiology*, the training program directors in that field declared, "While the USMLE Step 1 score is not designed to be used in resident selection, the lack of a reliable alternative makes this metric irreplaceable."

The more woke segments of the radiology community fought back. They worried that strict adherence to test scores would result in the near exclusion of African Americans from radiology training programs, given that they score on average about a standard deviation lower than White applicants. Clearly, equity in outcome mattered more to these people than did a superior performance. If eliminating ranked scoring meant a compromise in quality, so be it.

It is clear that marginal students are being admitted to medical school and that medical school curricula and assessments are designed to assure that all who matriculate will eventually graduate and achieve licensure. The question that arises is whether these revised standards in medical education will result in deleterious outcomes for the public. To answer this, we should have robust outcome measures in clinical care.

This is not easily accomplished. The variability that patients bring to the physician-patient interaction prevents reliable comparison among physicians. For example, a physician practicing in a referral hospital may deal with "sicker" patients with more comorbidities than a physician practicing in a community hospital. Often, the patient population factors into outcome rankings more than do the physician's skill and knowledge. Various grading systems have attempted to account for the variables that contribute to patient outcomes, but none has succeeded.

It has never been easy to assess physician competence. Over the years, many approaches have been tried, most notably written "recertification" examinations for physicians in practice for ten years, but none have stuck. Understandably, physicians have resisted periodic standardized testing. Their resistance makes it even more important to maintain the highest standards for medical training. Likewise, educators must be prepared to deny medical licensure to those who perform poorly in medical school and residency training. Current and planned policies, however, make uniform competence, let alone uniform excellence, an illusion.

Chapter 18

Millennial Coddling

In her bestselling book, *Generation Me*, Jean Twenge, a professor of psychology at San Diego State University, documents the narcissism and sense of entitlement that characterizes so much of the cohort of young people born between 1980 and 1996—*the millennials*. Said Twenge, "The purpose of school is for children to learn, not for them to feel good about themselves all the time." That wisdom holds for medical school as well. Although we don't yet give out participation trophies, we might as well.

To understand why the medical establishment has mollycoddled this generation of medical students and the one that follows—"Generation Z" as it is called—it helps to revisit the story of Libby Zion. In 1984, Libby Zion, an eighteen-year-old woman with a history of emotional problems, entered an emergency department in New York Hospital, one of the outstanding teaching hospitals in the United States.

Libby was on an antidepressant drug. Her complaint on admission to the ER appeared to be the flu, but she was noted to have neurologic symptoms as well. The newly minted physician trainees that routinely staff emergency departments treated her with a drug that could alleviate some of the jerky muscular movements they had noticed. They also gave her intravenous fluids to treat her apparent flu. A few hours later, Ms. Zion had a dramatic increase in her body temperature and developed a cardiac arrhythmia, followed by a cardiac arrest. She could not be resuscitated and died.

It turned out that a rare drug-drug interaction caused her tragic death. The two drugs were rarely given in combination, and the residents who prescribed the second drug were unaware of the interaction potential. Libby Zion's father was Sidney Zion, an influential lawyer and a columnist for the *New York Times*. He was convinced that the reason his daughter died was that the two residents were exhausted from their long night on duty. He subsequently won a highly publicized civil suit against the hospital and the physicians. More importantly, a law was passed that sharply reduced the time residents spend on duty during their training.

During the trial, experts pointed out that the drug interaction problem was so uncommon that most experienced physicians were unaware of it. In that pre-internet era, nothing could have been done to address that information void in an emergency setting. To satisfy the press and quiet the public uproar, however, hospitals could and did restrict duty hours for physicians.

Contemporary medical information systems dramatically reduce the risk of such medication errors. Physicians no longer need to consult print "formularies" each time they prescribe drugs. But the real legacy of the Libby Zion case is a dramatic reduction in the time available for the training of young physicians. Before 2003, physicians in training like me routinely worked between 112 and 128 hours per week. Today, the Common Program Requirements, the official policy of the Accreditation Council for Graduate Medical Education (ACGME), mandate an eighty-hour weekly limit, one day off in seven, and in-house "call" no more often than every three days.

Many studies have been conducted to test whether these restrictions were beneficial to either the trainees or the patients they served. The results are mixed. Residents claimed reduced stress and better sleep, but trainers registered concerns about less effective training. From their perspective, trainees had insufficient time to master technical procedures or the cognitive aspects of patient care.

Reduced hours also meant more physicians involved in each patient's care and more "handoffs" between trainees responsible for a given patient. Passing information between practitioners increases the opportunity for error. The more passes, the more opportunity—a sort of real-world replica of the parlor game, "telephone."

Recent studies published in the *New England Journal of Medicine* contend that relaxing some of the restrictions on the hours trainees can remain on a shift while maintaining the eighty-hour week maximum has not produced any negative consequences for trainees or patients. This may be true in the most sophisticated and wealthy academic medical centers, but whether it will hold true over time in more conventional settings remains to be seen.

The path from the Libby Zion case to current medical education is surprisingly linear. Medical students have assumed the psychological burdens under which physician trainees were said to work. These students now labor under the notion that the stress of medical practice is noxious, that the time demands are toxic, and that physicians are fragile and subject to "burnout." The very phrase "burnout" is problematic. We once associated that word with physicians who "burned out" after years of performing stressful tasks, after years of absorbing the repeated emotional shock of caring for suffering and dying patients.

In the new woke world of medical education, where almost everyone except the middle-aged White guy is a victim, students are almost encouraged to burn out simply for having to endure hard work, grading of any sort, and the occasional criticism. This is the equivalent of a soldier in boot camp claiming PTSD—and I suspect that is happening now as well. Dr. Christina Maslach, a professor of psychology at the University of California, Berkeley, has been a leader in the field of understanding and treating "burnout." Here is how she defines the phenomenon:

> A psychological syndrome emerging as a prolonged response to chronic interpersonal stressors on the job. The three key dimensions of this response are an overwhelming exhaustion, feelings of cynicism and detachment from the job, and a sense of ineffectiveness and lack of accomplishment.

From experience, I understand how busy clinicians might develop this syndrome if they are highly dedicated to their patients and feel defeated when patients do not respond well under their care. Of course, it is a luxury to be able to avoid such stress by working in a less demanding profession, which is just about every other profession. As much as I sympathize with the burned-out physician, I cannot extend that sympathy to medical students. Stress comes with the profession. If students cannot handle the minimal stress of school, they should not demand that the school reduce the stress level. They should seek a new profession.

A review of the topic by physicians from the David Geffen School of Medicine at UCLA and published in the journal *Clinical Teacher* in 2013 suggests that many young people may not be cut out for a medical career. The literature reveals that burnout is prevalent during medical school, with at least half of all medical students claiming to be affected by it during their medical education. More troubling still, studies show that burnout may persist beyond medical school and culminate in psychiatric disorders and suicidal ideation.

Unfortunately, medical educators have actively supported the idea that students are fragile. The designation "snowflake" did not come out of nowhere. Worse, they have convinced themselves that student burnout should be accepted as a legitimate diagnosis. In doing so, they have redefined a lack of resilience and personal discipline as something very much like an illness.

In my personal interactions with students, I have seen this collective resistance to personal accountability play out again and again. As noted previously, for several years, students have demanded that grades be eliminated in the preclinical years. They have especially objected to the reporting of grades to residency programs. God forbid that grades be used to establish class ranking or to determine which students garner honors designations. Students argue that since they were smart enough and motivated enough to gain admission, educators somehow demean them by monitoring their learning and academic efforts.

The students who perform well have an argument. Those who don't, don't. Today, there are simply more of the latter than there used to be. There is inevitably a large trailing "tail" to the normal distribution of grades. This tail represents the 9 percent of students who would have washed out fifty years ago. In the past, we knew and the students knew who made up that tail. Before the elimination of reported grades, many of those students saw the handwriting on the wall and dropped out. Today, there is no handwriting. These students may not even know how poorly they are performing and plod on as though all were well.

In a related argument, as a way of avoiding all traces of competition, students adopted the notion that teamwork was more important than individual achievement. Yes, teamwork is essential in health-care delivery, but every team needs a leader, and that leader should be the best-informed member of the team, the physician.

A third argument by the students at Penn, the weakest, was that "everyone else does it." The students surveyed at least twenty other medical schools to determine the grading policies at each. Sure enough, Penn was one of the last to yield to the policy of "pass/fail." Despite my objections, Penn surrendered. We did try to raise the passing grade to 75 percent on each exam. But using that metric would have produced too many failures and too much need for remediation. So we settled on 70 percent. Patients should hope that their physician was not one of those who scored in the 70 to 75 percent range.

Several of my students also suffered from a phobia introduced by millennials to America in much the way Cortés introduced the measles to Mexico—fear of the "microaggression." As an aside, doesn't the need to invent that word speak to the lack of real oppression in the lives of those who use it? How laughable that concept must seem to, say, the women of Afghanistan or the Christians in Nigeria or the ordinary citizens of North Korea.

It will surprise no one to learn that one of the most extraordinary breakouts of this mania occurred at a Harvard Medical School training site, the Brigham and Women's Hospital.

Widely admired, this powerful research center housed some of the best minds in American medicine. Among thinking people, that admiration dimmed considerably when the administration gave in to the student snowflakes on an impressively petty demand. They complained that the main auditorium made them "uncomfortable" because its walls were decorated by the portraits of former leaders of the institution, all of them chairmen of the department of medicine. These giants of American medicine did not own slaves, treat Indians poorly, experiment on Black patients, or help the American military in any way. Their sin was to be White, all of them, and, even worse, male. Their very existence was a microaggression. Upon realizing that history is not as racially malleable as, say, a TV commercial, the students demanded the removal of the portraits. As might be expected, the administration folded like Chamberlain at Munich.

Not to be outdone, my school, Penn, has launched a reexamination of the portraiture in the historic John Morgan Building and the Hospital of the University of Pennsylvania. I am willing to give odds on the conclusion Penn reaches.

What with all the competition, however muted, and the microaggressions, however minuscule, the entire medical workforce is now considered at risk of burnout. This has led to a new focus on "wellness" and concern for "work-life balance." As reasonable as these concepts might sound for, say, ad execs or attorneys, in medicine, they come at a cost.

Historically, physicians caring for patients with forms of cancer have made themselves available to their hospitalized patients, at least by phone, around the clock. The same has been true for general surgeons. Although many old-school physicians persist in this practice, many others, perhaps most, have retreated to group practices. For patients, this means that the point of contact is no longer *their* physician but the "physician on call." Shift work now focuses on the sickest and most acutely ill patients and is the dominant model in emergency departments and in-hospital acute care units. Other physicians increasingly prefer a nine-to-five schedule dealing with patients who are not acutely ill and mostly seeking preventive care.

Understandably, women physicians are typically more concerned with achieving work-life balance than their male counterparts. To the chagrin of Progressives everywhere, only females can give birth to children. Children take time to birth and to nurture. To criticize women for wanting time off would be to deny them their basic humanity.

That said, roughly 50 percent of new physicians are women. In real numbers, their graduation from medical school has more than doubled since 1980. Meanwhile, the number of men graduating has declined not just in percentage but in actual head count. In a 2019 *City Journal* article, Scott Yenor describes the consequences of this trend for patient care going forward:

> Though many women practice medicine full-time, most, according to a JAMA survey, ultimately work part-time or want to

shorten their hours. The survey—focused on recently graduated, thirtysomething doctors—found that 23 percent of female physicians worked part-time, compared with 4 percent of male doctors. Among doctors with children, 31 percent of females and 5 percent of males worked part-time. Even more tellingly, 64 percent of full-time female doctors have considered moving to part-time status, while only 21 percent of full-time male doctors have weighed the same option.

The net result of this trend will be less physician availability. One way to compensate would be to admit more medical students. But under current lax standards, increased admission would only lead to more poorly trained physicians.

That said, most physicians are dedicated to their patients and strong advocates for any interventions that enhance patient well-being. There is a danger that the respect the public holds for physicians, currently at a very high level because of the response to the pandemic, may not last. It depends on physicians adhering to the Hippocratic oath and putting their patients first. Medicine—millennials and Gen Zers take note—is not a profession for the overly sensitive, the easily stressed, or the flat-out lazy.

Chapter 19

The Woke Assault on Merit

Responding to the sorry state of medical education prior to the Flexner reforms, three academic physicians in Chicago created Alpha Omega Alpha in 1902. The society is the medical school equivalent of Phi Beta Kappa. Founder W. W. Root described the rationale behind its creation in a 1909 speech. "[…] this society is an honorary fraternity," said Root, "and membership is based exclusively upon scholarship, moral qualifications being satisfactory." Students were inducted into the society based on their grades and nothing more provided they maintained professional behavior. Even at its beginning, merit was all that counted.

In 1906, AOA amended its constitution to make clear its commitment to inclusivity: "Women are admitted on the same terms as men. In fact, race, color, creed, sex, and social standing form no barrier to membership, the only qualifications necessary being scholarship and character." In fact, it is hard to imagine any institution in 1906 that openly inclusive.

Traditionally, membership was limited to 15 percent of the medical school class. Over the years, membership became a key factor in determining a student's future career, as many of the most prestigious postgraduate training programs prided themselves on the number of AOA students in their midst. It was a seal of approval for the best and the brightest, regardless of "race, color, creed, sex, and social standing."

In much of the medical world today, alas, "merit" is considered an illusion, an unhelpful one at that. Consider the following mentions of the word or its derivatives in the AMA master plan [italics added]:

> The resulting differences in outcomes among historically marginalized and minoritized populations have been explained away through *the myth of meritocracy*. It is a narrative that attributes success or failure to individual abilities and merits. It does not address the centuries of unequal treatment that have intentionally robbed entire communities of the vital resources needed to thrive. (12)

> The health and non-health behaviors and choices provided to historically marginalized and minoritized communities and people arise from, and are shaped by, these conditions of deprivation and trauma, rather than causing them—as suggested by *the myth of meritocracy*, and *other malignant narratives*, that place the burden of responsibility for both harm and repair on oppressed populations. (19)

> *The myth of meritocracy* (36)

> The commonly held narrative of meritocracy is the idea that people are successful purely because of their individual effort, reflected in sayings such as "pull themselves

> up by their bootstraps" or "people just need to make better choices." The narrative is *powerful and harmful*. (37)

> Medical education has largely been based on such *flawed meritocratic ideals*, and it will take intentional focus and effort to recognize, review and revise this deeply flawed interpretation. (37)

These are the only references to "merit" in the AMA's eighty-six-page document. The authors understand that although equality of opportunity can coexist with meritocracy, "equity" cannot. Given the current atmosphere, AOA's unfortunate solution was to abandon academic merit based on measurable performance and to redefine achievement down. In May 2020, Dr. Richard Byyny, the current president of the AOA, writing in the journal *Academic Medicine*, showed himself a master of woke sophistry:

> "Scholastic achievement" refers to the qualities of becoming and being an excellent physician, such as knowledge, clinical care, patient care skills, competence, character, trust, trustworthiness, professionalism, communication and relationship skills, decision making, teamwork, lifelong learning, and leadership.

To this point, Dr. Byyny sounds like he is reading from the Boy Scouts handbook, but he was just warming up.

> Depending on the mission and goals of each medical school, "achievement in learning" could also include consideration of unequal barriers candidates faced at any level of education and in their personal lives, and how those were overcome. Measures of excellence vary

across the continuum of education, training, and practice. The choices of these measures are made by faculty and peers, professional organizations, state medical boards, patients, and colleagues. AΩA recognizes these assessments and evaluations in defining excellence as a physician and that they do, and should, evolve to reflect the values of the profession and evolution of assessment measures.

In sum, membership in AOA now means close to nothing. No longer can postgraduate residency programs depend on the AOA mark of excellence to denote the most academically talented students. The inductees may be pleasant, they may be "leaders," and they may have overcome barriers, real or imagined, but it is impossible to know if they really deserved acceptance by the AOA.

Sadly, the academic achievements of future inductees—and current members as well—will be diminished by the creation of nebulous categories like "leadership" and "unequal barriers." Defining scholastic achievement in terms that have nothing to do with scholarship degrades the language and cheapens the role of an academic honor society.

Many schools have eagerly adopted the new path to "scholastic achievement" as a mechanism to increase minority student induction into the honor society. For some, only an equal number of Black and White students selected for AOA membership will suffice. In 2017, Boatright and colleagues, as reported in the *Journal of the American Medical Association*, surveyed medical students applying for residency programs. They discovered that proportionately fewer Black students were inducted into AOA than Whites. In fact, Whites had a sixfold greater chance of induction into the honor society than Blacks.

The authors—no surprise here—called for better racial balancing. They refused to accept the idea that the imbalance might be because White inductees had done significantly better academically as measured by class rank and by scores on standardized exams. In a conclusion worthy of the Queen of Hearts, the authors argued that inducting more minority students into AOA could alleviate the deficit of minority faculty members as AOA membership is a characteristic of those hired as faculty. The authors do not seem to appreciate that faculty members were hired because of their talents. AOA membership was only a marker for achievement, not an achievement in itself.

Dr. Catherine Lucey, vice dean for education at UCSF, had her own bizarre explanation as to why few minority students qualify for AOA membership using traditional criteria. "Systems we use [for student evaluation] fail to take into account the extra work minorities are doing," Dr. Lucey told NPR. "[Minority] students have more stressors they have to deal with, low levels of racism that exist in our patients and our clinical environments." In addition to the imagined "stressors," Lucey somehow intuits that minority students have "extra work" and then implies that "extra work" makes these students more worthy of AOA membership. If extra work and stressors were the criteria, young women who give birth during medical school would be automatic inductees.

Penn Medicine took these recommendations to heart and decided to reduce the importance of class standing in determining AOA membership. As an alternative, the school formed a committee to develop a "holistic" evaluation. This would be acceptable if there were some way to acknowledge those students who are the actual academic elite, the ones who would benefit most from academically strong training programs. To promote equity of outcome, however, "reformers" have to slight the accomplishments of the most talented students. We hope the students selected for AOA membership were nice and helpful, but we *know* that some were not the most accomplished scholars. We know, too, that the original goal of the AOA founders has long been abandoned. For patients knowledgeable about medical education, finding an AOA certificate on the wall of a physician's office was once reassuring. No longer.

Penn's new process for selecting students for AOA election had its intended results. In 2021, 26 percent of the selectees were minorities while in previous years, minorities made up less than 10 percent of the cohort. Since AOA induction is limited to no more than 20 percent of the graduating class, some superior students were denied membership to be replaced by those whose claimed strength was engaging in more community activities. This was all unnecessary. Community-oriented students already had their own award system. It is called the Gold Humanism Honor Society. There was no need to downgrade AOA membership to celebrate the community activists.

Not surprisingly, most academics have supported the dilution of AOA membership. Here is a typical comment, this one from the leaders of the AOA chapter at the University of Michigan Medical School as noted in a 2020 entry in *Academic Medicine*:

> The AΩA national leadership team must take more definitive action to keep its chapters accountable for increasing UiM representation. A failure to do so will almost certainly lead to maintenance of the status quo, particularly among organizations not independently motivated to restructure their election processes. Ultimately, this inaction will continue to perpetuate inequality in AΩA elections.

If you're wondering, "UiM" means "underrepresented in medicine." It is not easy to keep up with the jargon designed to obscure academia's defiance of the "without regard to race, color, or creed" promise that drove the Civil Rights Movement. And so it goes—the honor society founded to identify inequality by honoring the most gifted students will now be tasked to eliminate "inequality" in AOA elections. Irony is not dead.

The American Society of Clinical Investigation (ASCI) was founded in 1908 to foster research into clinical medicine. Eligible for membership, according to the ASCI constitution, is "any physician residing in the United States or Canada who [...] has accomplished meritorious original investigation in the clinical or allied sciences of medicine [...]." Its leaders were the most eminent academic physicians of the time. Their goal was to create an elite organization to promote clinical investigation.

The ASCI continues to describe itself as "one of the oldest and most esteemed nonprofit honor societies of physician-scientists." By its own lights at least, membership comes in "recognition of a researcher's significant contributions, at a relatively young age, to the understanding of human disease." Many of its members, we are told, have been elected to the US National Academy of Sciences and the US National Academy of Medicine. Some have won the Nobel Prize and the Lasker Award, the medical equivalent of the Nobel.

Orwell had a word for the thought process in which leaders of these elite societies are currently engaged—doublethink, "the acceptance of or mental capacity to accept contrary opinions or beliefs at the same time, especially as a result of political indoctrination." In the spirit of doublethink, the ASCI has added a predictable wrinkle to its historic mission:

> To truly foster an inclusive ASCI and an equitable and diverse physician-scientist community, efforts are needed not just to diversify our membership and leadership, but to identify and mitigate racism and unconscious bias within our organization. With this goal at the forefront, the ASCI plans to establish a permanent Diversity, Inclusion, and Equity Committee through proposed amendment of the ASCI bylaws. This committee will be

charged with ensuring that the organization, its programs, and its mentoring mechanisms are free from racial and gender bias and promote and recognize diversity, inclusion, and equity. The committee will also be responsible for overseeing mentoring efforts that are focused on opportunities for underrepresented minorities.

As with membership in AOA for medical students, election to member status in the ASCI was a major boost to achieving tenure at the most prestigious American medical schools. That election demonstrated recognition by peers from outside one's home institution. For academic physicians, it was the *Good Housekeeping* seal of approval. Before the equity "reforms," the organization was purely devoted to merit. No one doubted that the 1.5 percent of its members who were "UiM" actually belonged in the American Society for Clinical Investigation.

Going forward, future UiM physicians will be tainted by the strong possibility that ASCI's diversity mandate influenced their selection. If these physician-scientists were, in fact, among the best and the brightest, no one will know. Most other ASCI members will suspect otherwise. The ASCI's abandonment of its elite heritage is not the least of its offenses against meaningful tradition. Most recently, the organization has vowed to forsake its nickname, the "Young Turks." To understand the absurdity of this decision, it is helpful to read the complete ASCI explanation:

> Coincident with the ASCI's founding in 1908, political reformists who became known as the "Young Turks" waged a successful revolution to replace the Ottoman monarchy with a constitutional government. The term came into idiomatic usage to describe those seeking to implement immediate transformative

change. The founding members of the ASCI took on this moniker in recognition of their rebellion against what they viewed as the antiquated practices and understanding of disease dominant at the time; they instead drew on advances in technology and knowledge of the underlying science, instituting as one of the organization's guiding principles "the correlation of science with the art of medical practice."

So far, so good. The phrase "Young Turks" continues to have the same metaphorical meaning as it did in 1908. Indeed, one of the most popular progressive TV shows is proudly named *The Young Turks*. The ASCI knows better:

> For the actual Young Turks, the revolution devolved. The group split into two main factions, one of which — known as the Three Pashas — bore responsibility for a campaign beginning in 1915 to exterminate the Armenian people (known as the Armenian Genocide; Meds Yeghern in Armenian) in which 1.5 million Armenians were deported, executed, or marched to their deaths. Continued use of the term Young Turks as a shorthand to describe the ASCI membership without contextualization of the atrocities committed under that name would risk causing hurt and offense. The ASCI Council and recently formed Diversity, Inclusion, and Equity Committee ask the membership to retire the term's use, instead emphasizing the spirit of scientific revolution from which it sprang and that remains true more than a century later.

Believe it or not, the leaders of the ASCI are very intelligent individuals. Yet they have decided to cancel the entire country of Turkey. Using the Armenian phrase for the Armenian genocide is a particularly deft touch. Apparently, we can use the term "Young Turks" only if we acknowledge the Armenian genocide at the same time. By this same logic, the Vikings, the Buccaneers, the Pirates, the Raiders, and a half dozen other sports franchises would have to change their names. Wokeness has descended into parody. Until about a week or so ago, no one who has ever used the phrase "Young Turks" felt the need to assure colleagues that they did not support the Armenian genocide.

The American College of Surgeons recently adopted a new approach to its membership and the college's role in society by adopting a commitment to anti-racism in all its functions. It is not clear if the leadership understands what this commitment means, but it aligns well with the war on meritocracy now underway in academia in general and in medicine in particular. The college issued a call in November 2020 to its members to develop an anti-racism perspective to the field of surgery and pledged that its leadership would "add [the value of] anti-racism to existing ACS [American College of Surgery] values."

Without intending, Dr. Bryan Leyva, a public health researcher at the University of Minnesota, highlighted the profound absurdity of this idea in a tweet to his thirteen thousand Twitter followers. Society should "abolish the meritocracy myth once and for all," he demanded. Not knowing enough to quit when he was ahead, Leyva added, "Idk [I don't know] who needs to hear this but scholarships, admission decisions, promotions, and awards based solely on meritocracy alone perpetuate social and racial inequality, and thus should be abolished."

Levya took particular delight in demeaning Dr. R. T. Bosshardt, who publicly resigned from his standing as a fellow of the American College of Surgery because of its new "anti-racism" stance. "All are laudable goals," said Dr. Bosshardt of the college's anti-racism initiatives, "but they have become poisoned with ideological meaning and taken primacy over other considerations, such as excellence, professionalism, competence, and compassion, which should be the overarching priorities in something like surgical practice." Bosshardt continued:

> Success in obtaining a residency position in any surgical specialty depends more on one's performance in medical school, recommendations from one's professors, and demonstrated dedication, such as taking a year to do research (as my daughter did to obtain an excellent residency in dermatology), than on gender, race, ethnicity, or some other identity. With medical school classes now 50% or more female and wide diversity in racial and ethnic composition, it is disingenuous to claim that our residencies and our College lack diversity or inclusiveness. Moreover, anyone who meets the requirements of Fellowship is welcome.

Dr. Bosshardt made too much sense for Dr. Leyva. Digging deep into his woke thesaurus, Leyva responded as follows: "This is what happens when toxic white fragility goes unchecked. White people start to believe their discomfort is justified and search for ways to fight back."

Missing from Dr. Leyva's thinking, but at the heart of Dr. Bosshardt's, is one essential variable: *the patient*. If we do away with all notions of merit and achievement, are patients to give up their right to seek the most accomplished physician? Patients expect excellence and professionalism from their physician, particularly a surgeon whose technique must be flawless.

In its arrogance, Leyva's position perfectly captures the absurdity of defending incompetence based on previous social disadvantages. No doubt society owes opportunity to all its citizens to achieve their potential. But medicine and surgery owe something else to patients—the highest level of skill possible. If the lack of a stable home environment prevents a young person from developing good study habits, should an unsuspecting patient be forced to compensate? The solution to disparate outcomes between White and Black students is not to ignore objective measures of academic achievement, productivity, and motivation, but rather to encourage the best and brightest to enter the profession of medicine and to demand the best of these students, "UiMs" included. Dr. Leyva's time at Brown University's Warren Alpert Medical School was noteworthy for his impact, as described by the school's office of diversity and inclusion:

> A native of Colombia who grew up in Central Falls, RI, Leyva knew he'd be one of the few Latino men at Warren Alpert Medical School. But he was caught off guard by how isolated he felt. "The fact that I wasn't represented in my faculty," he says, "and the fact that there weren't as many black or brown males in my class and in the classes after me—those things really, really affected me."

How many Colombians did the good doctor expect to find in medical school? "Fragility," apparently, does not seem to be reserved for White Americans.

Something else to consider: The research efforts of academic physicians require some form of extramural funding. The most important funding for research activities comes from the NIH and is historically based on merit. The amount of funding depends on funding requested by the investigator and available funds at the NIH. Typically, investigators submit grant applications and peer review determines whether funding is granted. Peers are physician-scientist volunteers who give a score to each application. Since only about 10 percent of grant applications are funded each year, competition is fierce, and the peer reviewers feel great pressure to dispense funds only for highly credible and useful research.

Even at the NIH, alas, merit is under assault. In 2019, writing in the journal *Science Advances*, Hoppe and colleagues, all members of the NIH administrative staff, observed that Black applicants for NIH funding are less likely than Whites to receive a rating for their applications strong enough to get funding.

The authors investigated all sorts of possibilities to account for these differences and came to the conclusion that Black researchers tend to pick topics that are not considered high priority by their peers—e.g., "racial and socioeconomic health disparities"—and tend not to have résumés as robust as those of their successful competitors. The solution the authors propose is reminiscent of the solution reached by the AOA honor society: just change the criteria for success. Hoppe and colleagues suggest that the NIH should intervene in the peer review process and direct funds to projects not considered to be high priorities by the peer reviewers if the grant proposals come from Black physicians.

It is not enough that the NIH has created specific programs to encourage minority applicants to receive funding and to help them develop their research programs. Now, the authors recommend corrupting the whole process so that Black scientists will receive funding even if their projects are considered inferior to the best research programs.

Progressives are demanding equal outcomes in research recognition not only for minorities but also for women. In a 2021 article in a publication of the *American Medical Association*, two researchers at Penn, Drs. Paula Chatterjee and Rachel Werner, pointed out that articles in the leading medical journals such as the *New England Journal of Medicine* and the *Annals of Internal Medicine* are less likely to cite articles in which women were the first or last authors of the cited article. This is yet another example of the way woke scientists seek out any disparity that might exist and then overtly or by innuendo attribute the disparity to discrimination.

This whole topic is highly complex. It centers on the way teams of scientists involved in research projects decide whose name is listed among the authors of a study and in which order. There are no hard and fast rules. Typically, the most senior, supervising scientist is listed last, and the researcher who did the most hands-on work is listed first. The fact that there are fewer women who head research laboratories merely reflects the fact that it is only relatively recently that women have pursued medical research careers in any numbers. Citation order is a lagging indicator of the current state of women performing medical research. The authors even point out that citations of women scientists have increased over the past twenty years by nearly 50 percent.

The other issue totally ignored by Chatterjee and Werner is the rationale for choosing a research paper to cite as part of a manuscript. I have published more than one hundred articles in the medical literature. The idea that I would pick a paper based on the sex of the first- or last-named author is absurd to the point of insulting. In fact, PubMed, the database of the National Library of Medicine used to find relevant articles, only lists authors by initials, not full names. Full names are revealed when one goes to the next step to pick a research paper to review. Like other researchers, I am more drawn to the status of the journal in which an article is published than the name of the author. Citing articles in the most authoritative journals helps establish the credibility of the research.

Chatterjee and Werner would have written a much fairer—though less provocative—article if they focused on which journals researchers cite. Instead, they trumpeted the disparity, however misleading, that they managed to uncover. In reality, the disparity does not reflect the bias, conscious or otherwise, of those citing articles. It reflects instead the lag in producing female investigators whose work merits publication in the most respected journals. As of yet, journal articles do not list the race of their authors. If they did, disparity hunters would have a brand-new way to waste everyone's time. Speaking of wasted time, Chatterjee and Werner reviewed more than five thousand articles.

Superficial as it is, the Chatterjee and Werner article inspired many of their fellow travelers to fret openly about the consequences of citation bias. A news item in the journal *Nature* shined a light on the phenomenon. "The paper is compelling because 'it shows just how much impact unconscious biases can have,'" said Reshma Jagsi, a female radiation oncologist and bioethicist at the University of Michigan. Jagsi argued that the disparity perpetuates gender inequity: Those whose work is promoted become leaders in their fields, and their work gets promoted all the more. We would surely undermine the quality of research if we tie a study's acceptance to the gender of the authors. In the process, we would also devalue the reputation of those women whose work deserves a citation.

It is of note that seven of the last eight department chairs at Penn's medical school have been women—at a university, by the way, whose president and provost are women. If Penn's "good ole boys" are restricting female career development, they have a funny way of showing it.

For the moment at least, NIH awards remain merit-based, but the same cannot be said for the intra-institutional ones. At Penn, a series of awards for clinical and academic achievement is granted to outstanding faculty. In the past, a committee reviewed award nominations based on such variables as meritorious conduct of clinical and basic research, mentoring of young scientists, and basic institutional citizenship. The review committee based its decisions on objective criteria focusing on meritorious work. No more. The new approach appears to acknowledge that previous awards were contaminated by the biases of past committees. From the announcement of the process for 2021:

> Penn Medicine is committed to promoting inclusion and diversity in its awards selection process. Recognizing that selections can be influenced by implicit biases around the

> gender, ancestry, ethnicity, and sexual orientation of candidates, the Selection Committee for each award grouping has been restructured to promote a diverse slate of nominations and awardees.

The only conclusion we can take from this mumbo jumbo is that, in the past, committee members rejected meritorious minority candidates because of racial prejudice. What an evidence-free insult this is to the faculty members who have served on those committees. At least four of the Penn awards are named for eminent Black physicians who served ably at the institution. Are we really expected to believe that previous committee members not only were racially biased but also were willing to exercise that bias by rejecting otherwise worthy applications? Can we cite at least one example, please?

Does it really matter if the next important research breakthrough is made by a Black physician-scientist? Does a scientist who has been to medical school and/or graduate school in biomedical science, one who has been mentored by senior faculty, really need an additional advantage just because of his or her skin color? What could possibly be the rationale for this other than the concept that diversity itself is more valuable than merit?

Black scientists today have every opportunity to conduct meritorious research. Indeed, many are among the best biomedical researchers. We do not improve the quality of federally funded research by expending NIH resources to meet racial quotas—excuse me, "goals." There is only so much money to go around. Funding is a zero-sum game. Besides corrupting the historic merit-based process, funding by race may be breaking the law.

Had the American Medical Association, historically a bastion of conservatism, stood its ground, these other institutions might have as well, but it did not. The AMA instead became a major funder of Progressive educational efforts and other leftist initiatives. The AMA recently published a "Declaration of Professional Responsibility" that asks physicians to "advocate for social, economic, educational, and political changes that ameliorate suffering and contribute to human well-being."

To understand the kind of "changes" a public organization really values, we need to look no further than its lobbying activities in Congress. The AMA, above all else, advocates for physician economic well-being. Its key legislative goals for 2020 include enhancing physician payment in Medicare, allowing physician-owned hospitals, advocating for insurance companies to maintain wide physician networks, and opposing the creation of a physician payment board empowered under the Affordable Care Act to review and modify Medicare payments to physicians. This old-school, bread-and-butter lobbying does not exactly square with the AMA's newfound commitment to all things equity.

The AMA does, however, go into righteous warrior mode in its advocacy for a new medical education paradigm. Specifically, the organization advocates for several unproven experimental initiatives with a particular focus on health equity issues. In one webinar, "Uprooting Racism Embedded in Medical Education," the AMA celebrates a program launched at the Warren Alpert Medical School of Brown University. As described by Dr. Paul George, the school's associate director of medical student education, he and his colleagues as well as a number of students decided to assess whether "lecturers were using race to depict a biologic construct rather than a social construct."

In medieval times, scholars debated how many angels could dance on the head of a pin. In modern times, the scholars at Brown did something equally useful. They examined every relevant lecture slide to decide, as a group, "whether race was being used appropriately or inappropriately." If used appropriately, it was allowed to stand. If used inappropriately, meaning race was depicted as a biologic construct, the group determined whether the biologic component was being taught explicitly or implicitly.

"When the lecturer used race as a biological construct, we did one of two things," wrote George. "We asked the lecturer to provide more context—so we asked them to think about race as a risk factor in terms of structural racism and how inequities in health care…and housing…and food…contributed to disease processes. Or if they could not do that, we requested that lecturers remove the slide entirely."

The ellipses, by the way, are George's. I guess…he was trying…to be…dramatic. His thinking, such as it is, nicely encapsulates the dilemma confronting physicians when dealing with racial issues. Without intending to, he showed how the demand to squeeze discussions of race into ridiculously narrow linguistic constructs can quickly lead to absurdity. One must marvel at the time wasted on this counterproductive nonsense.

Chapter 20

Genes Matter

As the good people at Brown made clear, young physicians acknowledge genetic disparities at their own risk. Much of the recent academic literature sends that message. One article after another stresses that physicians should assess racial disparities only in the context of racism and attendant social factors.

In a 2021 *New England Journal of Medicine* article, a team of authorities argued, "Most scholars in the biologic and social sciences converge on the view that racism shapes social experiences and has biologic consequences and that race is not a meaningful scientific construct in the absence of context."

Their argument is deeply problematic. In fact, a great deal of medical research suggests that individuals who self-identify as Black do manifest physiologic characteristics that cannot be ignored and cannot be attributed to social experiences. To this point, the very next week in the same publication, *New England Journal of Medicine*, a distinguished group of geneticists and epidemiologists identified very real genetic characteristics of African Americans that may convey a risk of disease:

Race, ethnicity, and ancestry have a complex and intertwined relationship that demands nuanced analyses. We believe that associations between race/ethnicity and disease outcomes should be interpreted carefully and that we should not assume that environmental, social, or genetic factors represent the only contributors to a given disease until causation has been proven. Conversely, we should avoid assuming that genetic causes have been ruled out, as this could undermine the discovery of genetic variants [...] variants that may partially explain increased prostate-cancer incidence among Black men.

In other words, it is wrong to deny the existence of race, and it is wrong to blame all disparities of an outcome on racism and its consequences. Race is a real entity and must be considered to properly care for patients of different racial categories, as imprecise as those formulations might be. Although our knowledge of the role genes play in disease outcomes is imperfect, there are too many proven examples of genetics as an important factor in racially disparate outcomes to ignore. Rejecting this evidence a priori is sheer folly.

Genetic differences do not imply genetic inferiority—far from it. In his study of Black athletic prowess, French researcher Jean-Philippe Leclaire discovered that "494 out of the 500 best-ever 100-metre sprint times are held by athletes primarily of West African origin." The fact that these sprinters came of age in a dozen different countries negates any argument that their dominance was due to environmental factors. Leclaire concluded finally, "Athletic performance is largely determined by genetics and specifically ACTN3, the so-called 'sprint gene.'" This gene is not found in "Black" athletes in general but preferentially in Black athletes with West African roots. As Leclaire observed, it has long been taboo in sports journalism to discuss biological differences. People have lost their jobs for pointing out the obvious. It is not quite taboo to speak of genetic differences in medical circles, but it is trending in that direction.

Although genetic traits may track with skin color, they are primarily due to geographic origins. One classic case in point is sickle cell anemia. This genetically transmitted blood disorder has everything to do with the regions in which mosquitos transmit malaria, predominantly sub-Saharan Africa. A genetic mutation gave people who lived in those regions—and their descendants—a higher resistance to malaria. Once removed from those areas, the sickle cell gene has no redeeming value. Those who inherit a certain abnormal gene from each parent live their lives at risk. In the last forty years, more than twenty-five thousand Americans died from the disease, virtually all of them Black. Even the most devoted CRT activists have shied from blaming this racial disparity on racism.

It was inevitable that the AMA's forays into advocacy would become entangled with the issue of race and racism. A recent example of racial advocacy appears to be a legitimate topic of medical concern but is, in fact, more about politics than about medicine. It concerns the observation that Black patients are disproportionately burdened by end-stage kidney disease.

Black patients make up nearly 50 percent of the patients on dialysis in the United States, four times their percentage of the population. The increased burden of kidney disease in African Americans, to a substantial degree, is the result of a gene originating in West Africa. For many years, however, it has been conventional wisdom to blame the disparate racial impact of kidney disease on substandard medical care in its many presumed mutations.

That disparity is due, at least in part, to African sleeping sickness, a lethal disease endemic to West Africa, the ancestral home of most African Americans. As can happen over many centuries when populations are exposed to a widely prevalent infectious disease, some individuals develop a spontaneous genetic mutation that gives them a unique resistance to that disease. In time, this mutation becomes more prevalent in the entire population as those fortunate to have the protection tend to live longer and have more offspring, who, too, are protected.

On the downside, the mutation that conveys protection against the parasite tends to amplify the kidney injury associated with conditions such as diabetes and hypertension. The combination of the two factors, the mutation plus the primary disorder, produces a much more severe form of kidney damage and a much higher risk of kidney failure. Despite claims to the contrary, the higher rate of kidney failure that Blacks suffer is not the simple result of the psychological stress of various forms of discrimination.

I am not suggesting that social conditions play no role in exacerbating kidney disease. What I am suggesting is that genetic characteristics, unique to people of West African descent, do play a role. It is a betrayal of the scientific method to attribute disparate health-care outcomes solely to social factors when genetic links are well established.

This betrayal seems willful when an investigator cannot identify a direct mechanism to connect the social factors and the disease in question. This is not to say that "stress" may not cause certain diseases and exacerbate others. Rather, the known existence of the genetic origins of some diseases shows the fallacy of assuming a racial/social explanation for any disease or all diseases.

Genetics, however, holds no interest for those whose primary goal is uncovering structural racism in the medical care of Black patients. Thirty years ago, a research study conducted under the auspices of the NIH sought to test whether modifying diets in patients with known kidney disease could slow the progression of their disease and improve kidney function.

To measure the potential benefit, the investigators realized that they needed a more precise method of measuring kidney function in the clinical setting than was available at that time.

Considering certain demographic factors like gender, age, and race in concert with a single blood test called "serum creatinine," they created an algebraic formula that gave a more precise approximation of kidney malfunction than previously available.

That study examined more than eight hundred patients, including several hundred Black patients. The study found that the formula had to be modified for Black patients: at any level of serum creatinine, White patients had a lower level of kidney function as registered on the GFR test than Black patients.

Over the next thirty years, other studies sought to improve the accuracy and reliability of the original formula to achieve an ever more accurate and consistent measure of kidney function. While multiple formulas were created, invariably a correction factor needed to be applied to give an accurate measure for Black patients as the results consistently showed the same discrepancy between Black and White patients as found in the initial study.

Until 2021, racially adjusted formulas served as the standard for reporting the level of kidney function. Millions of lab reports over the past twenty to thirty years have provided two results for kidney function. One applied to Black patients, and one applied to all others. Since race is not necessarily indicated in the lab request form, clinicians decided which value should be used with any given patient based on the physician's assessment of the patient's race.

In 2020, Nwamaka Eneanya and colleagues were the first to call for a rejection of the two formulas approach. They argued that a race-based designation was justified only under certain circumstances. One was that the use of the formulas conferred substantial benefits that could not be achieved through other feasible approaches. A second was that the use of race had to be transparent, and patients who rejected racial categorization had to be "accommodated fairly."

It was never clear what problem was solved by this proposal. Proponents constructed a scenario in which a clinician might delay a Black patient's eligibility for kidney transplantation based on the lab test result. Although technically possible, such an outcome was highly unlikely. Reformers failed to acknowledge that in real life, clinicians use many factors besides the specific GFR level to determine eligibility for kidney transplantation. Racial politics drove this change from the testing protocol, not any concern for the patient's health.

Dr. Eneayana's proposal led to the wholesale abandonment of a valuable clinical test in the name of political correctness. The American Society of Nephrology, the National Kidney Foundation, and many academic medical centers have announced that they will no longer support the separate reporting of the kidney function measure, GFR, for Black patients. The University of Pennsylvania Health System proudly announced this change as part of its efforts at "anti-racism." No need to ask why. That's just what a woke institution does.

The problem here is that in studies of thousands of patients, there is a difference between self-identifying Black patients and White patients. No philosophical musings about the nature of race can erase this observation. Those who wanted to abandon the race distinction argued that African Americans whose ancestors lived in East Africa differed from those whose ancestors originally lived in West Africa. True enough, but the ancestors of a vast majority of Black Americans hailed from a restricted region of West Africa. Individuals in this cohort share many common and distinct genetic characteristics, kidney function among them.

Experts like Dr. Andrew Levey and his colleagues, the original developers of the GFR formula, took to the pages of the *Clinical Journal of the American Society of Nephrology* to dispute the decision to abandon the race-based reporting. They correctly pointed out that there are robust data to support their position. Abandoning the race-based report, they argued, could deprive Black subjects of the opportunity to donate a kidney to a relative with end-stage kidney failure if the GFR test indicates previously undetected kidney disease. This could happen if a spuriously low value is reported because the formula used to calculate kidney function fails to account for the donor's race.

It is common in clinical medicine to review guidelines and laboratory testing standards periodically, but the decision to make changes has historically been based on new data or observations. This change in GFR reporting may be the first to be based on political considerations. The idea that Black patients have been injured in any way by the pre-George Floyd era reporting system is absurd. Evidence did not drive the decision to change. Fear did. Abandoning the previous system has already led to declarations by many organizations that they will avoid any other race-based formulas. I assume this will be the case even if the race-based formulas have life and death value.

There is another problem with abandoning the previous test algorithm. This coerced "reform" erodes the trust of Black patients. It implies that the previous approach was rooted in racial bias when it was simply based on rigorously obtained data.

The story ends with many thousands of dollars and many hours of valuable physician time devoted to forming a task force under the aegis of the American Society of Nephrology and the National Kidney Foundation. Task force members developed new formulas, reviewed all the old data, and found, well, nothing. The old formula worked fine. The new formula worked fine. Nothing will change except that the information will be reported differently.

Until new data refute previous observations, these efforts represent virtue signaling at its most potentially lethal. Most annoying is the idea that by adopting this new formula, the medical community was striking a blow against structural racism. Nonsense. This exercise was simply a cheap gesture that will change nothing. All it did was allow institutions to manifest their wokeness at the cost of considerable time and money.

Chapter 21

When Black Doctors Doctored

Harvard's Dr. Andrea Reid, about whom we spoke earlier, is a pioneer in a field that was best left unexplored. Her job at Harvard, according to *Harvard Medicine*, will be to eliminate systemic racism in medical education. She will undoubtedly succeed since there is no systemic problem to begin with. The world, however, would be much better served were she to invest her Harvard medical training in eliminating things that do exist such as cancer and the coronavirus.

Unfortunately, Reid's view of the ubiquity of medical racism resonates well with medical students at Harvard and has become a rallying cry for the new breed of woke physicians. Take the case of LaShyra "Lash" Nolen. On Twitter, Nolen describes herself as "a jubilant young woman on a mission to fight injustice through healing and education." As a first-year medical student at Harvard and president of the medical student government, Lash jumped right into the fray. In a *Boston Globe* interview, she demanded the renaming of the "Holmes" academic society because the person after whom it was named, Oliver Wendell Holmes Sr., "was a eugenist [sic], racist, and actively expelled the first 3 Black students to attend HMS." In fact, well ahead of the curve, Holmes admitted the three black students in 1850 and tried to admit a woman in 1847 but in both cases was overwhelmed by student and faculty opposition. It would take a century after Holmes's failed first effort before women were admitted.

Beyond these ignorant caricatures, the real-life Oliver Wendell Holmes was a renowned physician-reformer who saved thousands of women from death due to sepsis after childbirth through his advocacy of rigorous hygiene. He was a leading poet of his age as well. Unfortunately, Nolen's crude dismissal of Holmes's career is a symptom of her movement's—and her generation's—arrogant condescension to all things past.

Even before learning how to treat individuals, Ms. Nolen was learning how to cancel them. In the *Globe* interview, she unwittingly laid bare the foolishness overtaking medical education:

> […] I think physicians and health care providers should care about all things that affect their patients' health. There have been numerous studies that have come out and shown that access to housing, access to education, access to basic human needs are what folks need to have the best health outcomes. All of that is so inextricably connected to sociology and history and psychology. […] We can't continue to just stay in the realm of medicine, because our world gets the benefits from medicine.

"We can't continue to just stay in the realm of medicine"? Nolen barely entered that realm before deciding it was too small for her ambitions. In addition to confusing factors *associated* with poor health outcomes with factors that *cause* poor health outcomes, Nolen fails to appreciate the implications of her ideas for patient care. Her stated goal of becoming a surgeon conflicts with her "mission to fight injustice." An ER patient requiring emergency surgery cannot wait for Ms. Nolen to finish a protest march or write a naive op-ed. Being a surgeon is tough work. If Lash wants to become a good one, she damn well better "stay in the realm of medicine."

In the May 20, 2021, edition of the *New England Journal of Medicine*, Dr. Amanda Calhoun, an African American and self-identified "anti-racism educator," claimed that three high school students she was mentoring were uninterested in careers in medicine because, as one student wrote, "I think about the family members I've lost to the medical system [...]." Another wrote, "I really want to be a doctor, but I am terrified to be a patient." If these students take their cues from the media, who can blame them for being petrified?

Dr. Calhoun's essay is simply another attack on the medical establishment for the supposed "feelings" of certain medical practitioners. Without any evidence of a widespread series of practices that lead to poor outcomes, she proceeded to opine:

> We must identify the true pathophysiology of racial disparities: the racist, intentional oppression of Black Americans. Let's start training to identify the persistent mechanisms behind white supremacy: redlining, the school-to-prison pipeline, environmental racism.[36]

Historically, getting a paper published in the *New England Journal of Medicine* meant that you had made a new and important scientific observation. Now it means you are an African American physician who wants to repeat a bunch of clichés about past injustices and bring them into the medical school curriculum.

The essay evoked a few scathing responses from clinicians

---

36. Amanda Calhoun, "The Pathophysiology of Racial Disparities," *The New England Journal of Medicine* (May 20, 2021), https://www.nejm.org/doi/full/10.1056/NEJMpv2105339.

who had spent their careers treating Black patients and refused to accept such nonsense as "I've seen countless doctors roll their eyes at Black children in pain." Here is one brave response:

> [...] I am deeply offended by your inane remarks because I have been treating a large percentage of black Americans in my practice for decades. They are like family and are treated as such. I have never seen my colleagues treat black patients the way you describe as well, so please stop the activism and concentrate on healing instead of dividing.

The money, however, is in the dividing. Dr. Calhoun has her own website, amandajoymd.com, an unusual career move for a second-year psychiatry resident. The three specialties that she promotes on the home page are "Activist," "Innovator," and "Public Speaker." Under each of those specialties is a descriptive paragraph. In none of these paragraphs is either the word "patient" or the word "care." Dr. Calhoun claims to be "an outspoken advocate for justice and equality." As to patient care, that will apparently be left to White doctors. She, however, "helps organizations develop anti-racism curricula." My guess is that she doesn't volunteer.

As though it were needed, a new organization was recently formed to divert young woke physicians from the provision of care to the promotion of social justice. Abraham Flexner, the reader may recall, was the early twentieth-century reformer who modernized medical education. These people are so beyond Flexner they call their organization the "Beyond Flexner Alliance." BFA checks every woke and intersectional box on the planet.

According to the BFA, the alliance "aims to promote social mission in health professions education by networking learners, teachers, community leaders, health policy makers and their organizations to advance equity in education, research, service, policy, and practice." The website never says "or else," but that is implied. Scarier still, BFA is governed by many leading academic physicians and health-care leaders. To give some sense of BFA's scope and ambition, here are the topics covered in its 2021 Virtual Program:

- Championing **Equity**: programs that teach, model, measure, promote and reward health equity.

- **Diversity** now in Health Professions Education: race, ethnicity, gender, sexual orientation and gender identity, disability, culture, nationality, religion, and socioeconomic status among others and intersections of those identities.

- Innovations in **Learning Integration**: interprofessional education, integrated primary care, oral health, behavioral health, community integration and empowerment, social determinants of health, and health law among others.

- Moving to the **Quadruple Aim**: patient experience, population health, healthcare costs, and provider well-being in the context of social mission.

- Fixing the **Framework**: admissions, accreditation, post-graduate education, certification, hidden curriculum, payments, state and federal policies.

In reading this, I have to wonder how many hours of student and physician time will be squandered haggling over who gets what in the brave new world of intersectional medicine. What is clear is that care for the individual patient is not high on BFA's list of priorities. In any case, BFA is well funded by the Josiah Macy Jr. Foundation, the Robert Wood Johnson Foundation, and other funders who are either determined to reject the professional model outlined by Flexner a century ago or are afraid to stand in BFA's way.

Among other activities, BFA has created a survey so that medical schools can self-assess how woke they are and what areas they might expand to satisfy BFA's ambitious goals. If anyone wants to understand how the transformation of medical education is progressing, just spend some time "intersecting" with the Beyond Flexner Alliance website.

The focus on community health rather than on the scientific basis of medical care naturally leads to a commitment to understanding the social ills of communities. Once the leading medical institutions decided that racism explains disparate racial health outcomes, the natural next step was for physicians to concern themselves with understanding the social dynamics of the Black community. True, this project distracts physicians from focusing on the complex illnesses of individual Black patients. But no one at the BFA seems much concerned.

It bears repeating that the AMA, the BFA, and a dozen other powerful medical entities are now devoted to affirming the concept that the American health-care system suffers from systemic racism. The only cure for this scourge, of course, is the total transformation of medical school curricula. Once properly educated, future generations of physicians will be free of bias and racism and will finally provide the care that African Americans and other minority communities deserve. Unfortunately, this is all a myth, a lie actually, but one powerful enough to capture the attention of the academic establishment and a gullible, ignorant, and easily intimidated media.

In the real world, the world beyond "Beyond Flexner," academic medicine has been a bastion of meritocracy—defined as "the holding of power by people selected on the basis of their ability"—for a half century or more. This emphasis on merit has been a major strength of the system. It has made American medicine the envy of the world. Indeed, few other major systems, perhaps none, have been as free of racial or ethnic bias in promoting leadership and in recognizing individual achievements.

Of course, this has not always been true. In the early years of the twentieth century, medical educators were as blind to their prejudices against Blacks, Jews, and other minorities as were the leaders of just about every other American institution. By mid-century, in most of the United States, those prejudices had largely dissolved. I can cite any number of Black physicians who flourished in our meritocracy and whose achievements belie the idea that equality of opportunity is insufficient for Black physicians to prosper. If young Black doctors are serious about careers in medical care—and not medical activism—they should look to those physicians who accomplished greatness when racism wasn't just "structural" but was in your face.

Take the case of Dr. Ed Cooper, the Norman Roosevelt and Elizabeth Meriwether McLure professor of medicine at the University of Pennsylvania. Born in Jim Crow South Carolina nearly forty years before the passage of the Civil Rights Act, Dr. Cooper completed his internship and medical residency at Philadelphia General Hospital (PGH). He then served for two years as chief of the US Air Force General Hospital in the Philippines. Upon leaving the service, he went on to complete a National Heart Institute Fellowship at PGH and joined the hospital's staff and the faculty of the University of Pennsylvania School of Medicine (UPSM) in 1958, several years before the term "affirmative action" was coined, let alone applied.

Among his leadership roles at PGH, Dr. Cooper was president of the medical staff, chief of the medical service, and cofounder of the Stroke Research Center. Widely published, Dr. Cooper served extensively in national and local organizations. He chaired the committee that produced the American Heart Association's (AHA's) scientific statement "Cardiovascular Disease and Stroke in African American and Other Racial Minorities." In

1992, he became the first black president of the AHA. His many awards include the AHA's highest honor, the Gold Heart Award. In his late nineties, as I write, Dr. Cooper was a brilliant clinician, an admired leader, and a beloved teacher. The fact that he self-identifies as an African American had nothing to do with his achievement and the respect with which he is held at the University of Pennsylvania.

Gerald Thomson, MD, is the Samuel Lambert professor emeritus of medicine and the Robert Sonneborn professor emeritus of medicine at Vagelos College of Physicians and Surgeons (VP&S) at Columbia University. Born in Harlem to Jamaican parents, Thomson chose to attend Howard University's medical school because, as a former Red Cap at Grand Central Terminal, he could commute between Washington and New York for free. Thomson completed his residency and fellowship training in nephrology at State University of New York's Downstate Medical Center/Kings County Hospital in Brooklyn long before anyone thought to demand shorter hours and competition-free assessments. In 1970, he was recruited to join the Columbia University faculty.

During his forty-eight years as a member of that faculty, Dr. Thomson served as a clinician, a teacher, and director of a maintenance dialysis program. He also has been an advocate for justice and human rights in health care, director of medicine at Harlem Hospital Center, chief medical officer and executive vice president for professional affairs at the former Columbia Presbyterian Medical Center, senior associate dean at what is now VP&S, chair of the American Board of Internal Medicine, and president of the American College of Physicians.

An activist in his own right, Dr. Thomson devoted his energies to those areas in which a physician's knowledge makes a difference, most notably addressing and remediating the disparities between the care provided at public and private hospitals. Dr. Thompson, now retired, was a brilliant clinician, an admired leader, and a beloved teacher. The fact that he self-identifies as an

African American had nothing to do with his achievement and the respect with which he is held at the Vagelos College of Physicians and Surgeons at Columbia University.

In 1994, the American Medical Association named Dr. Lonnie Bristow, an internist from San Pablo, California, as president, the first African American so designated. "This is a day of firsts," said the sixty-five-year-old Bristow upon his selection. "I am not unaware that I will be the first specialty candidate, and the first African-American ever to head America's most prestigious medical organization." He added, "However, neither fact will define my term in office."

Raised in Harlem by a minister father and a nurse mother, Dr. Bristow attended Morehouse College in Atlanta as a sixteen-year-old and dabbled on the side as a varsity quarterback. After a four-year stint in the newly integrated US Navy, he finished his undergraduate degree at CCNY and his medical degree at NYU, all without the aid of any equity-inspired preferences. From New York, he headed to California, MD in hand, and began a practice in the San Francisco Bay Area specializing in job-related injuries and illnesses.

It was not until 1968 that Dr. Bristow could receive full membership in the AMA. A full century earlier, 1868 to be precise, the AMA debated the issue of race and gender integration but deferred the decision-making to local chapters. Finally in 1968, in response to concerted pressure from civil rights organizations, the AMA finally rejected racial discrimination within its ranks and allowed Black physicians unqualified membership. In 1981, the American Society of Internal Medicine elected Dr. Bristow its first Black president. Other honors soon followed. Upon being elected to head the AMA in 1994, he said not a word about racial equity, let alone climate change. "My greatest concern," he said, "is to see that the doctor-patient relationship is protected in the health-care transition." The fact that he self-identifies as an African American had nothing to do with his achievement and the respect with which Dr. Bristow is held in the State of California.

A generation younger than Doctors Thomson, Cooper, and Bristow, Dr. Ben Carson could have been diverted from his drive for excellence by the sinecures increasingly available to minority physicians. Instead, Dr. Carson took the road less traveled by, and that, as Robert Frost reminds us, "made all the difference."

Living with his single mom in Detroit, the young Ben attended a largely black public high school and did well enough to receive a full scholarship to Yale. From Yale, Dr. Carson entered medical school at the University of Michigan. Although he initially struggled, he responded to his low grades—they still graded then—by outworking his fellow students. He soon began to excel and was accepted by the Johns Hopkins University School of Medicine neurosurgery program. There he served one year as a surgical intern and five years as a neurosurgery resident. He completed his final year as chief resident in 1983.

Freed from worrying about racial equity or climate change, Dr. Carson was able to focus on one of the most demanding of specialties, pediatric neurosurgery. In 1987, Dr. Carson made the news when he served as the lead neurosurgeon in a first-of-its-kind operation—separating twins joined at the back of the head. At age sixty-two, Dr. Carson retired from Johns Hopkins School of Medicine at the top of his game. A social activist in his own right, he now had the clout and the time to have a real impact on society, making a credible run for president in 2016 and serving under President Trump as secretary of housing and urban development. The fact that Dr. Carson self-identifies as an African American had nothing to do with his achievement and the respect with which he is held at Johns Hopkins and in the nation at large.

As the historical record makes clear, the breakthroughs made by Doctors Cooper, Bristow, and Thomson make the idea of "systemic" racism, even in the 1950s, suspect. They were all inducted into Alpha Omega Alpha at a time when the criteria were simply scholarship and "satisfactory" morals. These great men did not need dubious new categories to enter an academic honor society.

By the 1990s, Dr. Carson's success at Johns Hopkins and Dr. Bristow's election as head of the AMA render the accusation of systemic racism absurd. Despite these examples of Black physicians rising to the very highest levels of academic medicine and leadership roles in the most influential institutions, current leaders of academic medicine, in a willing burst of amnesia, declare that "systemic racism" taints us to this day.

In an example close to home, Dr. Meghan Lane-Fall, a professor and chair of the medical faculty senate, asked attendees at a June 2020 kneel-down for "Black Minneapolis resident George Floyd" to acknowledge that racism haunts the halls of power at Penn. Not coincidentally, Dr. Meghan Lane-Fall serves as vice-chair of inclusion, diversity, and equity for the department of anesthesiology and critical care (each department now has its own watchdog). "Racism threatens our science, clinical practice, and our education," the good doctor insisted. She also expressed hope "that we can embrace the discomfort that these conversations will bring…." From her perspective, "Prioritizing comfort over action undermines our mission."

Lane-Fall felt free to extrapolate from Floyd's death that the "system" of academic medicine, and medicine in general, is racist. Sorry to disappoint you, doctor, but American medicine has not manifested any hint of widespread racism since the advent of the modern civil rights era.

Of course, this does not mean that no one associated with medicine harbors biases. It does mean that Black physicians have more than ample opportunities to achieve their full potential as they have had for at least the past half century. The achievements of Drs. Cooper, Thompson, Carson, and Bristow certainly suggest as much.

Chapter 22

Back to the Future

In a 2019 editorial in the *American Journal of Medicine*, William Frishman, chairman emeritus of the Department of Medicine at New York Medical College, said out loud what many of us are thinking:

> Medicine in the United States today is a true meritocracy, and we have come a long way to remove discrimination and to improve inclusion. Medicine needs to remain a meritocracy. We can still fine-tune the profession, but in the process, let's not eliminate awards and honors. Excellence needs to be recognized, as it encourages progress. We are all better physicians because of it, and in the end, society benefits. Let's keep the Nobel Prize.

As Dr. Frishman attests, not everyone has given up. Not everyone is okay with woke hegemony. There may be a way to end that hegemony, but there is no easy way. The medical establishment from top to bottom is thoroughly infected. The desire of students to pursue a medical career will persist and so will the desire of Progressives to recruit an army of social justice activists. Too many people are invested in the disease to welcome a cure.

To reverse the current trajectory will take a shock to the system. This might take the form of a financial shock that no one will enjoy or a court-ordered shock that the Progressives will resist or, ideally, a system-wide recognition that woke medicine is slowly killing the people it is supposed to help.

When that moment comes, if it comes, reformers must be ready. Fortunately, a working model already exists. The future, I would suggest, lies in the past—not in the way-back past that constricted opportunities for women and minorities, but in the recent past that welcomed everyone but coddled no one. It is time for a neo-traditional counterrevolution, one that is as focused and as forceful as the woke revolution now laying waste to American medicine.

As neo-traditionalists, we might begin by demanding students spend more time on scientific education. This added time will come at the expense of the time-wasting social justice content in the curriculum, but that's as it was and should be. A two-year science curriculum would allow topics such as normal physiology, the molecular basis of disease, pharmacology, biomedical statistics, medical imaging, and other advanced topics to be reintroduced into the curriculum in a more robust fashion.

Again, the time for these expanded topics could be secured by eliminating the current, foolish components of many medical school curricula. I refer here not just to the race-baiting courses but to feel-good practices, such as having first-year students spend several hours each week in medical clinics before they have even the most basic understanding of medical care.

The latter practice is particularly counterproductive. It is based on the notion that students who have spent years trying to gain admission to medical school now need rudimentary exposure to patients to understand the rationale for learning the scientific material needed to be an effective physician. It's like *Sesame Street* for doctors.

"Active learning" for medical students makes great sense, but the current time spent on each topic is too limited to be effective. While it is true that faculty members decide what should be taught, the administration decides how much time should be allowed for each component. That is the problem. Educators should abandon the pretense that learning in medical school is best accomplished by methods associated with adult learning theory.

Unlike students in other disciplines, medical students cannot define the subject matter they need to learn. It is the faculty's responsibility to decide the content and the detail of medical education. Students complaining of too much science and too little clinical training should not dictate terms. These students obviously fail to understand that science underlies clinical learning and makes sense of it.

There is no question that standards in medical education are substantially lower than in previous decades. Expensive coaching programs provided by medical schools do not solve that problem. They enable it. We should demand their elimination. We should also eliminate ongoing assistance such as school-provided tutoring for students who cannot master the curriculum. No student has a *right* to finish medical school, but they do have a responsibility to perform in an exemplary fashion. If they cannot, they should leave.

Medical-related fields such as nursing and pharmacy have a higher attrition rate than medical schools. It is bad enough to finesse students through high school. It is downright dangerous to finesse them through medical school. Low attrition rates are the problem, not high ones. Given that medical schools continue to reduce the requirements for admission, the only guarantees of competence are high standards for granting an MD degree.

Reduced requirements for admission are, of course, closely related to the push for student diversity. This reduction leads inevitably to lowered standards for graduation for everyone. There is no good reason *not* to raise standards to where they were in the recent past. To suggest Black students cannot meet those standards is to engage in what George W. Bush called "the soft bigotry of low expectations."

The historic presumption had been that anyone who successfully passed the requirements for admission should be able to complete medical school. This was the justification for passing almost everyone who matriculated. If, however, the admission requirements remain diluted, the standards must be raised. The surest way to do so is to raise the passing grade on exams, allow only one remediated exam if a student fails, and require evidence of the student's ability to think beyond his lecture notes. The last of these three will show the student's capacity for independent learning. Multiple-choice exams have their value—especially for the graders—but free-text answers do a better job of showing mastery of complex issues.

The initiatives to increase diversity should not compromise the quality of the students in medical school. There is no compelling evidence that more Black physicians will improve the health of the Black community. The only goal of medical training should be to optimize the health of the patients. If there is a need for physicians to practice in minority communities, economic incentives work a whole lot better—and with less injustice to the Constitution—than does the recruitment of physicians based on skin color. Any college student who wants to be a physician should have the opportunity based on the student's intellectual capabilities, character, and nothing else.

We should insist that merit be rewarded in medical school as it was not too long ago. We should insist that class rankings be maintained and reported to residency programs to guarantee that the most accomplished students train at the most advanced programs. A return to merit will allow patients and institutions to easily identify the most accomplished practitioners.

The public should have some assurance that superior credentials are based on superior performance. Patients who decide to seek treatment for their cancer at topflight programs, such as the MD Anderson Cancer Center or Memorial Sloan Kettering Cancer Center, expect their clinicians to be the best and brightest. Those institutions need mechanisms to identify outstanding young physicians. In fact, all academic medical centers need those mechanisms.

We should pressure honor societies to honor merit and give students and faculty incentives to perform in an exemplary fashion. Criteria for membership in those societies should once again be academic achievement, not community activism, as is now increasingly the case.

Researching outcome disparity for Black patients makes sense but not if done obsessively as it is now. Importantly, too, researchers must check their biases at the door and once again use scientific rigor in the design and execution of their studies. More and more observational studies aiming to prove discrimination simply because there is a disparate outcome have led to a dead end. Routinely, these studies fail to incorporate the perspective of the patients and physicians involved. Often, researchers don't even inquire.

We should lean on journal editors to stop publishing studies whose authors set ideological ground rules—critical race theory, anyone?—for assessing the results of the study. Journalists who cover these stories should seek out and report dissenting views from established scientists, not just confirming ones. If they don't, they should hear from us.

We should persuade scientific journals such as the *New England Journal of Medicine and the Journal of the American Medical Association* to stop enabling racial paranoia by publishing opinion pieces from activists whose complaints can never be proven. These journals squander their scientific credibility by promoting racialist views of society and the medical community. They need to stop dabbling in Progressive journalism and start presenting only cutting-edge scientific information once again.

Allowing angry minority physicians in training to spout their unsubstantiated racialist nonsense is wrong and should have ceased yesterday.

Academic medical centers can do much to improve the medical care of minority communities. Whether they can improve the health of these communities remains to be proven. Medical care would be improved by enhancing access to care. Lack of access is driven by economics and not bias.

If academic medical centers want to improve Black lives, they should open spacious and well-staffed outpatient facilities in inner-city neighborhoods in addition to the multimillion-dollar units placed in affluent suburbs. It may be cheaper, of course, to launch highly publicized, virtue signaling, anti-racist campaigns, but I suspect most Black patients would prefer good outpatient care to good intentions.

There is room in the medical establishment for at least one medical school to renounce identity politics and return to a demanding and rigorous four-year curriculum grounded in hard science and quantitative analyses of the biochemical basis of disease. There are students, thousands of them, who would rather focus on hard science than on soft-core Marxism. Great book curricula have their adherents in some liberal arts colleges. A similar restoration of rigor in medical education would generate a dedicated following. This won't happen by accident. We need to make it happen.

Abraham Flexner completely upended medical education in the early twentieth century. His study revealed a widespread lack of scientific rigor and the failure of medical school curricula to incorporate new scientific knowledge. We need a new Flexner. We need someone willing to take the woke goggles off and look at medical student preparedness as it exists. The new Flexner needs to be independent of the accrediting agencies that have encouraged the current mess. This new Flexner cannot be indebted to the medical school administrations that have, for too long, gone along to get along.

Abraham Flexner was not a physician. Paradoxically, this independence allowed him to perform the radical surgery that the system then needed. We need to establish a new, independent Flexner commission, one that is immune to the threats of cancel culture, one that will root woke ideology out of the medical establishment and save American medicine from itself.

For this to happen, we all need to stop being afraid.

About the Author

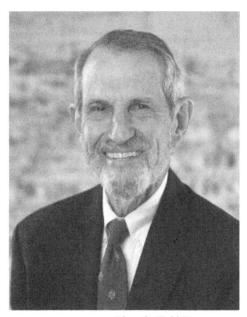

Photo by Todd Zimmerman

Stanley Goldfarb has been an academic physician for the past fifty years with broad experience in research, education, and patient care. He has served as editor of medical journals, interim chair of the Department of Medicine at the University of Pennsylvania Perelman School of Medicine, and most recently, as Associate Dean of Curriculum at Penn.

Made in the USA
Las Vegas, NV
06 September 2023

77156407R10125